TIRZAH HAWKINS BCHHP

Overcoming Autoimmune

Discover the ROOT CAUSE of your health conditions and how to heal from them 100% naturally.

Be blessed.
Tirzah Hawkins

First published by Natural Health Warriors Books 2020

Copyright © 2020 by Tirzah Hawkins BCHHP

All rights reserved. No part of this publication may be reproduced, stored or transmitted in any form or by any means, electronic, mechanical, photocopying, recording, scanning, or otherwise without written permission from the publisher. It is illegal to copy this book, post it to a website, or distribute it by any other means without permission.

Tirzah Hawkins BCHHP has no responsibility for the persistence or accuracy of URLs for external or third-party Internet Websites referred to in this publication and does not guarantee that any content on such Websites is, or will remain, accurate or appropriate.

Designations used by companies to distinguish their products are often claimed as trademarks. All brand names and product names used in this book and on its cover are trade names, service marks, trademarks and registered trademarks of their respective owners. The publishers and the book are not associated with any product or vendor mentioned in this book. None of the companies referenced within the book have endorsed the book.

First edition

ISBN: 9781674158068

This book was professionally typeset on Reedsy.
Find out more at reedsy.com

For my husband, Daniel
Who always believes in me.

Contents

Foreword	iii
Preface	vii
How to use this book.	1
Will this work for me?	5
Early Signs of Autoimmune	11
Programs, not Remedies	16
What will it take for you to commit to yourself?	21
My Journey	24
Losing weight the easy way.	32
Basics of Health	36
Natural Health is Preventative	36
What direction is your health heading?	37
Germ Theory vs Terrain Theory	38
Healthy Plants and Animals	41
Digestion	42
Intestines and Antibiotics	44
Four Organs of Elimination	45
Two causes of disease	48
Some Basic Body Needs	52
Getting Started: The A B C Method	61
Do you want to be healed?	61
Activate: Opening the pathways	65
Activate: Elevated Emotions	71
Activate: Emotional Clearing	76
30 Day Change Anything Challenge	86
Brainstorming	87

The Process	88
Build: Providing the tools	111
Cleanse: What does this mean?	118
Cleanse: getting out the "bugs"	122
Your Personal Consultation	125
General Information	126
Occupation and Recreation	142
Mental Health	145
Diet	151
Different Diet Types	159
Medical History and Conditions	162
Personal and Home Care Products	168
Summary	172
A 30 Day Food List	174
Food list	174
Thank You	180
Also by Tirzah Hawkins BCHHP	181

Foreword

If you are reading this book, it is likely that you, or someone you love, has some form of autoimmune condition or autoimmune symptoms. Off the top of my head, I can think of at least a dozen people very close to me who have a diagnosed disease or suspect that they have one, and they are struggling with some form of symptoms every day. Here's the thing that doctors don't tell you; you CAN actually fix it. Not patch it or mask it with a prescription, but actually dig down to the core of the cause and correct it, naturally and safely. This book might be the spark to ignite your fire of healing.

I have a strong family history of autoimmune, and honestly, always assumed I would end up with one myself. I have have been married for over 14 years with five children, ranging from ages 2 to 11 years old and thought myself to be decently healthy, in spite of a few seemingly minor symptoms here and there.

After kiddo number 4, I started having increasingly worsening symptoms that was ultimately triggered by a Tdap vaccine given following a bad cut. I developed highly sensitive food allergies and significant neurological issues affecting my vision, balance, mental clarity, and more. By the time I had my fifth child, some intensely stressful life situations left me physically and emotionally a mess and I felt like I was falling apart.

At one year postpartum, I felt no more recovered from childbirth than I had a month after I had my baby. I was constantly bone deep exhausted. The doctor wanted me on thyroid medication for hypothyroid symptoms. My hair was falling out. Seasonal allergies left me miserable. I could not lose the baby weight. My skin was a mess with painful acne and rosacea. Brain fog left me struggling to function. I had headaches and migraines almost daily. I was barely going through the motions of life and somehow trying to raise a family.

I didn't know what to try next.

Now, I am a researcher naturally, not by trade. If I am going to buy an appliance or pair of shoes, you better believe I am going to read all the reviews and compare everything out there to try and get the best that I can.

In trying to heal my symptoms over the years, I have read articles and books on how to help your thyroid; heal acne and rosacea; alkalize your body; get rid of migraines; this diet and that diet... You get the picture. Sometimes, something would seem to help for a short while, but nothing really fixed anything. Despite my best efforts with my research, I knew there had to be more to figuring out the problem, and I wanted to get to the root of it so I could actually heal.

"The journey of a thousand miles begins with a single step" Lao-Tzu

I started working with Tirzah with cautious optimism. She asked more questions than any doctor ever did, and these little details about my health gave a picture that showed how my symptoms now are actually the culmination of many years of my gut not functioning optimally.

I figured that if this can help with something at all, then it was better than trying nothing because I had nothing to lose. Little did I know that it would quite literally change my life. My goal was to try and gain some energy, lose some weight, and clear up my skin.

Within the first few months I began having symptoms disappear. The dreaded headaches went away. Weight started to drop and my hair started to fill in. But that was only the beginning.

As I began to learn more about how our body works and natural health in general, my fascination grew and I realized just how little I actually understood. I started to soak up as much information as I could and began to see more how incredibly complex yet beautiful of a puzzle our body's healing process is.

In all of my previous reading of how to fix X, Y, or Z, I was only looking at a piece or two of a very large puzzle. Tirzah introduced me to the fact that this puzzle is essentially the same in every person. We might have different pieces, but they essentially fit together the same. But how do we put this together now to fix the problem that is seemingly unfixable?

There is a right and wrong way to do many things. You don't put your shoes on before your socks. You can't paint the house before you put up the siding and prep it. Natural health, also, has a process and order to healing. The root cause of ill health is the same and the general route to heal is the same, but there are countless possibilities of tools that our body needs to complete the journey.

This book and Tirzah's program will help guide you through the process to select the right tool at the right time to enable you to take charge of your health and healing. Her passion for healing and helping others comes through, and it is just as personal for her as it is for you.

In the past year and a half, I have had almost all of my neurological problems disappear. This is one of the most amazing and unexpected improvements for me. I can take my little girls on the merry go round with all the lights flashing at night and experience absolutely no dizziness. Two years ago, I couldn't even look at a merry go round without getting very dizzy and off balance. If we took our children to the fair, I would walk with my head down and block the lights and movement of the rides from my view.

My eyes aren't crossing anymore and my vision is stable. I very rarely get headaches. My food allergies and sensitivities are significantly less sensitive, and I have been able to reintroduce some foods that I could not have even a trace of previously. I am not exhausted all the time. My hair has grown back. I am much happier with my weight and my ability to maintain it. I have many small moles all over my body continuing to fade and disappear (a sign of liver improving).

I applied much of my new-found knowledge to my family and have been able to improve my family's health as well. (Goodbye asthma inhaler and allergy medicine!) My journey is still ongoing and I look forward to see where I am in another year.

The solution to overcoming autoimmune is not a simple one where you simply take a pill and, poof, you are healed. It is a multi-faceted natural approach that takes dedication, lifestyle change and consistency to see true results. It is an investment in your long term health.

Is it worth it? Absolutely, yes! Tirzah's extensive knowledge of natural health and unfailing optimism and support have been absolutely critical in every step of my journey with her.

I highly recommend Overcoming Autoimmune and hope that it helps you regain your life and health the way it has for me.

Rebekah Homutoff

Preface

Disclaimer

As a natural health practitioner, I (Tirzah Hawkins) do not examine, diagnose or treat, or offer to treat or cure or attempt to cure, any mental or physical disease, disorder or illness. As a drug-free practitioner, I do not recommend or prescribe or recommend changing the dosage or discontinuing any prescription medications or pharmaceutical drugs.

1

How to use this book.

This book is meant to read like a conversation as if you were sitting across a desk from me during a private consultation. This is not a reference book. For the most part, it is meant to be read from cover to cover, over and over, again and again. There is a lot of information contained here, but don't let that overwhelm you. With each rereading, you will be able to absorb new information, understand something that didn't make sense the previous time, and with application, begin to change your health dramatically.

After working with clients for over seven years, I realized how much I had to review the same information with every single person. Even someone who enjoys natural health and studies it as a hobby to better their health and that of their family is missing this basic understanding of how their body works.

I talk with many people on nearly a weekly basis who still struggle with their symptoms in spite of working with a traditional naturopath. These people find success in alleviating their symptoms naturally that isn't much better than what they would accomplish with a Western medicine doctor.

Naturopaths are crippled with the regulation of their profession by the federal government. In 18 states now, in order to license as a naturopathic doctor, natural health professionals are required to study Western medicine techniques and methodology. When they finish their schooling, their practice becomes a muddy blend of herbal and prescription medicine.

A true natural health professional should always be talking with their clients about the "cause" of the symptoms instead of how to only address or mask the symptoms. The 1800s herbalist Samuel Thomson said, "Remove the cause and the effect will cease."

When we only look at one part of the body, we miss how the rest of the body affects that part. If you have a thyroid disorder, you end up only looking at the thyroid and miss how the digestive or intestinal system may be playing a role in the weakness of that organ.

"But I don't have digestive symptoms. And my bowel movements are normal." I hear that from people time and time again. When I begin to ask them questions related to their digestion and intestinal system, that you'll find in the consultation section of the book, they realize how many signs and symptoms they were missing.

Western medicine teaches us to look at the body in parts. That's why we have pulmonologists, gastroenterologists, podiatrists, cardiologists, and all the other "-ists" you can think of. This approach is limited because you can only bandaid a certain organ or system when you aren't looking for the actual cause of the symptom.

My Methodology

This book comes out of my own experience with drastically changing my health, combined with over eight years of natural health schooling, and seven years of working with clients.

First, it talks about my own journey of struggling with health issues the majority of my life. Then I share some stories from clients I have worked with.

As I continue on in my journey, I keep learning newer or better ways of getting to the core issue and removing it.

I don't focus on symptom relief. Many of you reading this may get hung up on this aspect. "Well, what about my thyroid? How does this correct the lack of hormones there?

What about my heart? How does this reduce my risk of POTS? Strokes?

Heart disease?

I have multiple autoimmune conditions. How does what you are saying apply to all of them?"

Throughout my studies, I have never been interested in the symptoms. When you go to a Western medicine doctor, you are looking for symptom relief. Yes, there are herbs that can provide symptom relief. I may mention a few here. I provide that information to make your journey to true health easier and more comfortable.

However, I am much more interested in looking at what is causing the symptoms than just relieving them. When we focus on symptom relief, we need a bandaid for each one. For a lot of people that I have worked with, that could be 10-20 different things. If we focus on just symptom relief then there is no energy or money left over to address the cause. But if we can focus on the cause, then the symptoms will go away. I will repeat that concept multiple times throughout this book as it is important to understand in order to truly recover.

For example, you put your hand on a hot stove and leave it there. It hurts, so you call up a Western medicine doctor and ask what to do.

"What are your symptoms?" the doctor asks?

"Well, I have terrible burning pain and some blisters forming," you reply.

"I'll prescribe you an ointment you can put on that should help both the blisters and the pain."

You try the ointment, applying it to as much of your hand as you can, but the pain still increases. You call the doctor back. "Doctor, the pain is still increasing."

"I can prescribe you a pain-relieving drug you can take orally."

You try the medication which takes the edge off enough that you can function a little and go about your day. But you and the doctor never discussed the cause of the burning and pain.

Contrast that with calling a natural health professional. They'll ask enough questions until they figure out that you are still keeping your hand on the hot stove. After they have gotten you to remove it, will they then talk about something for the pain and blisters.

We need to get to the root of the issue and not merely look at the symptoms.

Inflammation is one of the things at the core of most of the problems associated with autoimmune diseases. It's like a slow-burning fire.

Imagine a small fire in your living room. It smolders away and creates a lot of smoke, making it difficult to breathe. You call your doctor and say that you can't quit coughing and have tightness in your chest. Your doctor prescribes a cough suppressant and maybe a muscle relaxer.

By evening, the smoke has set off every alarm in your house. This keeps you awake that night.

You call your doctor and mention difficulty sleeping for which they recommend a sleep aid. The smoke in your house begins to darken your skin. The doctor prescribes a whitening cream.

As the fire eats away at your house, it causes a hole in your ceiling. You call roofers to repair the hole. Now your carpets need to be replaced. And your furniture. Eventually, your whole house is destroyed, and you are left wondering what went wrong? You did everything the experts said. But, you didn't get to the cause of the problem. A good natural health professional would have told you from the beginning to go get your fire extinguisher and put the fire out before moving on to address the coughing caused by the smoke.

I hope that this helps you to see the difference between addressing the symptom(s) and addressing the cause(s).

2

Will this work for me?

Your autoimmune disease is not any more special than anyone else's. People like to exclude themselves. When I announced this book or my Natural Health Warriors program, I had many people ask, "Will it work for what I have?"

Autoimmune diseases all have the same core cause. Since our bodies are different and each of us has our own strengths and weaknesses, there is probably an unlimited number of ways that autoimmune diseases can show themselves.

All of the information in the book applies to you and each of your conditions, whether they have a label or not, so don't exclude yourself if you are honestly looking for a solution.

It was Henry Ford who said, "Whether you think you can, or think you can't, you're right."

Have you heard of the placebo effect? This is a phrase that demonstrates the ability of the mind to influence the body. If someone believes something will make them better, then it will. And if someone believes that they cannot get better, then no miracle in the world can help them. This is why certain people die of cancer within a few months of getting a fatal diagnosis.

We have all heard stories of people receiving a doctor's diagnosis and being given a few months to live, only to continue living for years. Or about people being injured in a car accident so severely that they were told they would never walk again, but yet they go on to later run marathons. How can some people overcome such extreme physical conditions and injuries?

Our body has an innate ability to heal itself. Nothing I can give you will heal you. Nothing a doctor gives you can heal you. Your body was designed to do all the work itself. It just needs the right tools and support.

Right now, each minute, your body is creating millions of new cells to replace the billions that are used and destroyed throughout your body on a daily basis. The purpose of this is to get rid of those that are not functioning properly and to make new, healthier cells.

Where this beautiful process goes wrong is when we are missing a vital ingredient for the cell or when something gets in the way.

Missing a vital ingredient is called a deficiency.

Think about all the components of your house. When your house was built, I'm sure you wanted it to start with a strong foundation. Then a framework was put up. We want that framework filled in with insulation and covered on the inside and out by different ingredients to create a strong, secure structure. There is usually a finishing siding put on the outside and the inside walls are finished with sheetrock and paint. We hope that our roof is sturdy and protected with tar paper and shingles.

We'd like our kitchen to contain a sink, refrigerator, drawers with knobs or handles, etc. Walk into any home improvement store and look at the vast array of materials that go into making a house.

We'd like our house equipped with a way to heat and cool itself. Running water and electricity are taken for granted as well as waste disposal and niceties such as a couch to sit on and a tv to watch.

That sounds complicated, but our body has so many more components and vital parts than a house.

What Building Materials Are You Providing?

Think about the way you eat as providing materials for your body to build itself. The best building materials come from a wide variety of organically raised fruits and vegetables harvested in their season and grown in quality soil that was adjusted to provide the nutrients for each plant grown in it. Our body benefits from the complete proteins found in pasture-raised animal meat. We can't forget the fruits of the sea that provide essential fatty acids which we affectionately call omegas.

These are the nutrients that provide the support to the core components of the body's house, giving it a strong foundation, walls, ceiling, etc.

The rest of the things we eat that don't provide highly nutritional benefits, such as delicious biscuits and gravy, are just our comforts: our television set, a comfy couch or a soft bed. These don't contribute to the core structure or function.

If your body is constantly repairing little weak spots in its ceilings, walls, or foundation, but all you are providing it to build with is televisions and couches, how effective is that process going to be?

How sturdy will your foundation be? How waterproof your ceiling? How windproof your walls? We wonder why our house struggles to function for us as we desire when it is lacking what it needs in order to properly do that.

Things That Get in the Way

The second reason why your body can't make a healthy cell is that something is getting in the way. This is called toxicity and the culprits are called toxins.

Our body can become overrun by such things as viruses, harmful bacteria, yeasts and fungi, parasites, and heavy metals.

Imagine trying to repair a wall where a hive of bees has made its home without ever getting rid of the bees. Or preparing healthy food in a kitchen that has been overrun with ants and cockroaches. How about trying to wash yourself in a bathroom that is never cleaned. How excited would you be to live in this house?

When we don't address toxins and remove them from the body, these conditions can build up and overrun the body, preventing it from being able to correct itself.

Just as it requires some effort on our part to facilitate a hive of bees being removed from our house, in the same way, our body requires some effort on our part for keeping these toxins, that can't ever be fully eliminated from our lives, at a healthy minimum.

Desire, Belief, Determination, and a Comprehensive Program

There is no single solution for these issues. Overcoming them requires desire, belief, determination, and a comprehensive plan or program.

Now, I can help you with some of the things you'll need for optimal health, but I can't give you desire. I can tell you what is possible, or what I believe is possible. I can tell you what I've accomplished in my own life and some of the amazing things my clients have accomplished. But I can't make you want to change. I can't want this for you more than you want it for yourself. And I want it for you badly. It's why I continue to study natural health. I've already accomplished an immensely better level of health for myself which continues to improve as I continue to study. But I want to find even better ways of helping my clients. It's why I'll continue to put out new programs, new courses, and new books. I very badly want you to achieve a level of health that is beyond what you believe is possible right now.

I can't make you want it. So this book is dedicated to those people who want it for themselves more than I want it for them.

Now I can help you with belief if you are willing. As you begin to apply, actually apply, and not just read, the information in this book to your life, you will start to get some little wins. As those victories accumulate, you'll get brief glimpses into what is possible. As you recognize those wins, you'll begin to believe bigger and better things are achievable for yourself. All you need to do is start with an open mind. Be open to achieving better health than you ever thought was possible.

Determination is your responsibility. It is different from will-power. We have a finite amount of willpower available to us each day. Now we can definitely cultivate more will-power, but that isn't always a very fun process. I can personally attest to that with my experience of many different diet plans over the past two decades. But will-power is not important to this process. In fact, I try to take will-power as much out of this material as possible.

Determination is about never giving up. It's deciding that you can have this vibrant health and energy I'm talking about, and that you will do whatever it takes to achieve this until it is yours. It makes you look for different ways of doing things. When will-power fails, determination makes you try again. But rather than just trying to strong-arm it with will-power, determination helps you take a step back and think: what can I do to make this easier for myself? What can I do to apply this differently? What is a different way of doing this that would accomplish the same end result? How can I help myself be more successful?

Determination means never giving up on your goals. My husband started smoking at the age of fourteen. He spent the next fourteen trying to quit. The first seven years of our marriage contained one failed attempt to quit smoking after another. At times, he failed many weeks in a row. Sometimes he took a reprieve from fighting.

Did I ever encourage him to quit trying? Not once. I knew the more times he tried to quit, the more likely he was to succeed. He only failed if he quit trying.

He was determined to quit smoking. The key was that he didn't try the same thing over and over. He tried many different techniques, giving each a solid effort: cold turkey, gum, nicotine gum, nicotine patches, the Allen Carr book "The Easy Way to Quit Smoking" method, limiting it to the weekends, and many more. Finally, he discovered BecomeAnEx.org. The community on that website provided the support he needed to finally quit smoking.

The information in this book is most likely completely different from anything you have heard or tried before. I'm hoping it will be that "new thing" you are looking for

The way that I can help you to become more determined is to help you realize your worth. You are worthy of reaching your goals. I believe that vibrant health and energy is a birthright that everyone deserves.

My goal is to help you find your worth: to stop putting yourself and your goals last. You can't help someone else achieve their goals and potential if you aren't willing to achieve yours.

Have you ever flown on a plane? As the plane is taking off, the flight attendants instruct everyone, in case of emergency, put on your own oxygen mask before you assist anyone else.

We all create our own emergencies every day. We will all be much more effective at helping and caring for one another if we have our own oxygen masks on.

Finally, you need a comprehensive plan, a program, to follow. This book is not written for someone who wants to take a little bit from here and a little bit from there. Each tool I introduce to you works to make the others stronger. In fact, the one that seems the most ridiculous to you is probably the one you need to focus on the most.

It's definitely okay to start with just one thing. In fact, you will probably be more successful if you do. Start with one thing and master it. When you can continue it without much difficulty, then incorporate another tool.

Some people will be able to incorporate everything in this book at once, run with it, and have a completely different body and feeling of health in one year.

Not everyone is a rabbit. If you are a tortoise, don't compare yourself to a rabbit. Take it slow. You'll have many improvements as you go. Within a couple of years, you too will look back at the day that you bought this book and not recognize the person you were then. The pain and struggle you were in at that time will just be a memory.

Hold that vision and let's move forward.

3

Early Signs of Autoimmune

Autoimmune diseases are really myriad in number and symptoms, but they all stem from the same root causes. People try to disqualify themselves thinking that what I am suggesting could never work for them. Just take a look at the list of warning signs. This information applies to you if you are experiencing one or more of the symptoms on the list.

There are quite a few early warning signs for autoimmune disease. I've seen some of these show up in client's children as early as one year of age. I see more and more people talking about it in even younger children as time goes on.

One of the very earliest warning signs is gastrointestinal issues. Any sign of improper digestion or elimination should be thought of as a warning.

What are some signs of improper digestion? Burping or bloating after meals. Acid reflux or heartburn. Food sits heavy after eating. The stomach doesn't feel like it empties very quickly.

What are some signs of improper elimination? Foul-smelling intestinal gas or stools. Not having a bowel movement for each meal eaten (one train into the station, one train out). Hard stools. Stools that float. Stools that don't maintain their form. An insufficient quantity of stool passed each day. For someone eating three meals a day, they should be passing an amount of stool equivalent to the length of their arm each day.

Those are the very earliest warning signs. If we would just address these as soon as they start, which for some people are early childhood, then we could head off a whole host of health issues. I don't remember who said, "May you never know the disease you prevent," but the advice is sound.

Many of us are taught to disregard these warnings. Western medicine teaches us that as long as we are having regular bowel movements, which for some people may be as few or fewer than once a week, then that is "normal" for you.

This is some of the most dangerous advice I've ever heard. Constipation kills. Besides that, it is extremely uncomfortable and creates a huge energy sap.

One of my experiences with natural health was progressing from two to three bowel movements a week to one or two a day. My energy levels soared within days of maintaining that.

Getting our basic body functions like digestion and elimination on track does wonders for our health. It is a core foundation for moving away from disease and towards health.

Most of my clients come to me with much more advanced conditions. Had they started working with me sooner, it would be much easier and faster to achieve what they are looking for.

The sad thing is that, especially in America, we are taught to ignore our health until it bothers us enough that we want a change. And even then, we only look to cover the symptoms.

A friend of mine has visited China several times and has experienced regions where they pay their doctors to keep them healthy. As long as they remain in vibrant health, they pay their doctor. If they were to develop an illness, the doctor would no longer be paid.

Can you imagine that? How many of your current doctors would you be paying right now if their job was to keep you healthy?

I'm sure my definition of health and yours varies widely. It is important that we are on the same page as we move forward.

The World Health Organization has defined health as "a state of complete physical, mental and social well-being and not merely the absence of disease or infirmity."

That is the definition of health that I want you to keep in mind as you continue to read this book. Someone who is living in a state of unhappiness is not healthy no matter how few physical symptoms they may have. The lack of mental well-being can lead to physical repercussions down the road.

My goal is to help you achieve this all-encompassing level of health. As you read, you will notice that some of the exercises, chapters, or supplements are meant to address your mental or social well-being. I hope that as you work through these, you will realize how interlaced with your physical health these components are.

Starting early and more advanced conditions

The sooner that you begin to notice any symptoms such as the ones we've already mentioned in regards to digestion and elimination and the ones I will mention here shortly, the easier it is to achieve and maintain health.

Those who are the closest to health when they begin working with a natural health practitioner will make the quickest progress.

As someone acquires more and more symptoms, their body actually slows down: physically and emotionally. This may be why emotional and physical issues are so interlinked. Negative emotions can slow body processes down to a point that they don't sustain healthy life. Each affects the other in a vicious cycle.

Another issue resulting from this "slowing down" is the creation of an environment very hospitable to undesirables such as viruses, bad bacteria, parasites, yeasts, and fungi.

Water illustrates this point very clearly. Which has more algae, scum, and mosquitos in it: a flowing river or a stagnant pond? When things flow and move, they stay much cleaner and aren't a ready home for parasites. When things stagnate, they become a breeding ground for a multitude of microorganisms, many of which are harmful to the body.

The following is a list of common signs of advancing autoimmune conditions in the body. The more of them that you have and the longer that you have allowed them to progress, the more difficult they may be to overcome.

This doesn't mean that it is impossible. It will just take a longer duration of time and effort according to how long you have had the symptoms; more nutrients and supplements will be necessary to address the cause and to provide symptomatic relief if desired in the meantime.

- acid reflux
- acne
- ADD/ADHD
- allergies
- Alzheimer's
- anxiety
- arthritis
- asthma
- B12 deficiency
- blood clots
- blood sugar imbalance
- brain fog
- cardiovascular disease
- chronic congestion
- dark circles under eyes
- depression
- digestive issues: (gas, bloating, indigestion, constipation, diarrhea, reflux, heartburn
- dry eyes
- fatigue
- fibrocystic breasts
- frequent illness
- gallstones
- hair loss
- headaches
- intestinal spasms
- joint pain
- mood swings
- muscle pain
- obesity
- pancreatitis
- PMS symptoms
- poor concentration
- sinus issues
- skin issues: acne, eczema, psoriasis, rosacea
- sleep problems, apnea, insomnia
- swollen, reddened, or painful joints
- uterine fibroid

All of the symptoms above can be controlled and eliminated through the processes revealed in this book.

In fact, I've seen many other issues clear up as well. Rebekah, who wrote the forward and has worked with me closely for a year and a half at the time of this publication (Jan 2020), had extreme vertigo and other vision and neurological issues that were not being improved by working with a neurologist. As we worked on eliminating the cause of her autoimmune conditions, the neurological issues cleared up as well.

It is amazing what the body can heal itself from. Even conditions where permanent damage was thought to have occurred have been healed by the body's amazing regenerative abilities.

Your body has the knowledge and ability to repair broken bones! Keep that in mind the next time you think healing isn't possible for you.

If the body wasn't made to heal itself, you would have every bruise, scrape, cut, fracture, and broken bone that ever occurred in your life. We would all be walking around looking like a zombie out of a horror movie.

The body has amazing regenerative abilities when we provide it with the tools, resources, and the care it needs and help it eliminate the wastes and toxins that get in the way.

Key Learnings

We need to address the body as a whole.

"Remove the cause and the effect will cease." - Samuel Thomson

If you have any of the warning signs, this information applies to you.

"Whether you think you can, or think you can't, you're right." Henry Ford

Your body has an innate ability to health itself.

Your body requires a lot of different nutrients for its structure and function.

Proper waste and toxin removal are essential.

The journey to health requires desire, belief, determination, and a comprehensive program.

There are many advance warning signs and symptoms for autoimmune.

The sooner you start working to repair your health, the easier and faster it will be.

Write down in a journal any other key points you would like to remember before you continue reading.

4

Programs, not Remedies

Have you ever walked into a health store and asked, "What do you have for this____?" (Insert hot flashes, bladder infection, trouble sleeping, warts, pain, or any other symptom you have experienced.)

I'll admit that I was guilty of that, too. We've been trained to look for patches or remedies for our ailments.

When we go to the doctor, they often have a neat little single prescription they can give you that addresses your problem. We all know that there are herbs that can do what prescriptions do that are safer and easier on the body.

We often walk into herbs shop and treat it as a natural doctor's office looking for the "prescription" that we need. But when we do this, we are often limiting natural health to just a "bandaid" when it can be so much more powerful.

We also have the approach that we should take one dose of the "prescribed" herb and Woah, notice a huge difference. That isn't how herbs work.

When something creates a dramatic difference in your body in just one dose, as many chemical prescriptions do, it is often working against the body. It is stopping some sort of normal body function in order for you to notice a dramatic difference so quickly.

Let me let you in on a little-known secret: your body is always trying to keep you alive and keep you healthy. When we have symptoms, it's because something is getting in the way of or missing in order for the body to function in a normal healthy way. This symptom can often be uncomfortable especially because it isn't the way the body was made to function. But it is what the body is reduced to doing because it hasn't been given everything it needs.

When we take a prescription, we stop that normal body function that is trying to keep us alive and trying to protect our vital organs.

Think about somebody who has a skin condition like athlete's foot, psoriasis, eczema, or acne. It doesn't commonly occur on the trunk of the body. Instead, it is pushed to the extremities: the top of the head, the arms and hands, the legs and feet.

The body needs to drive the offending toxin from the core of the body and away from the vital organs. It pushes it away and out.

If we go and get a prescription steroid cream to stop the issue in one place, the body is forced to create another pathway to keep the toxins away from vital organs. We haven't solved the problem nor supported the body.

If you have ants in your kitchen, and you block the current hole they are using, they will just find another way in, maybe multiple ways in. The results may be immediate, but there are long-term ramifications. The problem was not solved.

When you use something to kill the ants that they can take back to their home, you are addressing the issue and have found a long-term solution.

This is the difference between working with your body and working against it. Working against it will create overnight results with long-term ramifications. Working with it takes a little longer, but the results are better and longer-lasting.

When we begin to take herbs to address these issues, change doesn't happen overnight. Instead, the herbs begin to work with the body to address the issue.

Let's reflect on the Chinese again. They have one of the oldest systems of natural medicine in the world and believe from millennia of experience that fast medicine is bad medicine and slow medicine is the best medicine.

In our fast-paced society, we want quick solutions, but those aren't always the best, especially in herbal medicine.

Yes, I expect my clients to begin to feel improvements almost immediately. Those who are following a full supplement regimen with a healthy diet and lifestyle plan should notice a difference in their health within just a week or so of beginning.

However, the issues that they have had the longest will take the longest to see improvements in. They are more deep-seated. The body has created multiple ways around those issues because of it trying to survive that has to be rectified.

You can't give up early. You have to give the healthy changes the time for your body to heal and resolve each issue. A good rule of thumb is it takes one month of dedicated following of the program for each year that you have had the issue.

But you have to be committed. Each "cheat" sets you back a couple of days. If you "cheat" two or three times in a week, you have just nullified any forward progress you may have made that week.

This is where people get frustrated. We think of programs, diets, regimens, and anything similar as a restriction, as a form of slavery of ourselves almost. That is why we reward ourselves when we do something good for ourselves.

"I just worked out for 45 minutes. I can have a donut." Right there, we just nullified the workout. It would almost be better to only workout for 15 minutes and not have the donut.

This mentality that it is difficult to eat and be healthy is why we have to do emotional work as well. When we can address that mentality, we can make the process easier.

Addressing the root

It can be dangerous when we try to just control symptoms and don't address the root. There are two women I know who struggled with urinary tract issues, but the bladder and urinary pain was actually a warning sign of a greater issue.

One of them was Jennifer. She was constantly struggling with urinary tract pain. She came to me asking what she could take for it as she had been on antibiotics numerous times in the past year, and I was cautioning her about the damage the antibiotics were causing to her immune system.

There is an herbal formula I recommended to her that contains goldenseal, uva ursi, parsley, juniper, and a few other herbs. I also suggested the use of probiotics.

Jennifer would take the herbal formula for a week or so whenever she had painful urinary issues. She would be consistent with the probiotics for a little while longer. But she wasn't making the lifestyle changes that would support whole-body health. She wasn't taking enough supplements to help her body clean out and repair from years of damage.

Her pattern continued like this for a year or so, where she would have painful urinary issues and take the herbal formula every few months. She was controlling the symptoms but doing nothing to address what could be causing the pain.

Typically the herbal formula would provide relief from the supposed urinary issue within 24 hours, but one time it didn't. Jennifer said it was even making the pain worse. When the pain continued to increase, Jennifer went to the hospital where they discovered she had some uterine cysts burst. If we had addressed the lifestyle issues causing the pain instead of just the symptoms, we would have been able to help her body eliminate and stop producing the cysts.

Essential Oils

I love essential oils. They have become increasingly popular in the past two decades. However, essential oils are limited in what they can do in helping your body overcome autoimmune conditions because essential oils are not a good source of nutrition.

Your body needs vitamins, minerals, antioxidants, amino acids, essential fatty acids, and other nutrients found in foods and herbs.

Essential oils are not foods. In fact, I rarely recommend them to be used internally at all. These are extremely potent substances that should be used with care to prevent injury, internally and externally.

You can get the same benefit from using essential oils by mixing them with a carrier oil and applying them to your skin, especially the soles of your feet, along the spine and the back of the head.

When I'm working with someone with autoimmune symptoms, essential oils will not be a high priority as part of their supplement plan unless I think it will be helpful in improving their emotions.

When it comes to a balanced supplement plan, essential oils are like decorative icing on the cake. They are not part of the core components.

Key Learnings

Natural health is more powerful when we address the whole body and not just the symptoms.

The body can't heal overnight from deep-seated issues. We need to make a long-term commitment and be consistent.

Addressing only the symptoms can allow other issues to go on unchecked.

Essential oils are helpful but not essential to helping autoimmune conditions.

Write down any other thoughts or reflections you had about the chapter in your journal.

5

What will it take for you to commit to yourself?

My husband has a podcast called "Your One Shot". The concept around it is really important, in my opinion, for people to get.

We have one life here on earth? Why aren't we focused on it being as happy and joyful and enjoyable as possible? When we do, we actually contribute to other's happiness, joy, and enjoyment.

There is enough here on earth for all of us to experience the fulfillment of our lives. When we live our purpose, which is what brings us fulfillment, we are able to give more to others.

In this country, we take owning a vehicle for granted. And if it breaks down, we can usually get another, often for very inexpensive.

What if, at the beginning of your life, you were given one vehicle and that was all that you could ever own for the rest of your life?

Would you drive it as much as possible? Or would you find alternative ways of transportation in order to make your vehicle last as long as it could?

Would you provide your only vehicle with regular maintenance or would you neglect the care of it?

When the engine light comes on would you ignore it or seek to get it fixed as quickly as possible?

We use our bodies for much more than we use the vehicles that transport us throughout our lives. The vast majority of people I come in contact with don't take the time to value, care for, or listen to their bodies.

Your body uses all the engine lights and alarm sounds that it can. Whenever we experience a symptom we don't like, that is the body's way of getting louder.

Very few of us use the intuition that comes naturally to us. It's the still, small way that our body uses to communicate with us. When we don't listen, the body has to resort to harsher and louder ways of getting our attention.

I also encourage people to think twice before having body parts removed. We think that it's the easy fix to just have an organ or a gland cut out.

The circumstances in the body that caused that part of you to start giving you trouble still exist even after you remove the part that was screaming for your attention.

The condition that creates gallstones still exists after you remove the gallbladder. Without your gallbladder, you will have a more difficult time digesting fats and need to take an enzyme formula containing lipase whenever you eat more than a gram or two of fats.

The condition that causes your tonsils to become inflamed every few months still exists in the body even after you remove them. The tonsils are a gateway for the immune system. Without them, the body is susceptible to deeper and more severe infections.

Even the appendix is now being shown to play an important role in the health of the body.

We aren't made with spare parts.

Instead of just cutting them out, we need to seek to understand what is going wrong in the body and how can we correct it.

Let's start giving the body the daily, weekly, monthly and seasonal maintenance it needs. You will notice a dramatic difference in your health.

Key Learnings

Removing an inflamed body part does not correct the condition in the body that caused the inflammation.

Our body requires maintenance if we want it to be healthy and in good working condition.

Write down anything else you wish to remember from this chapter.

6

My Journey

"Look at the size of that baby!" Those were the words my mother heard frequently in the hours and days after my birth while I was still in the hospital.

Her room was just down the hall from the baby viewing window. When I was born, there was only myself and one other baby in the hospital. It was a premie, and I was a giant by comparison.

Even at ten pounds, three and a half ounces, I was my mom's easiest delivery. Most of the difficulty with me was during pregnancy.

I guess I wasn't too much trouble the first 18 months or so of my life. But before I was two years old, I was no longer the chubby little baby. Instead, I was extremely skinny and underweight as I was allergic to every food she tried to feed me.

Because of my severe allergies, she would puree me a single fruit for breakfast, a vegetable for lunch, and a protein for dinner. I then had to have that food rotated out of my diet for five days.

This continued on for a few months.

Just a few years before, my mother had become a Christian. There was a church meeting one night during these difficult months of my life. She took me to it and had me prayed for.

Then she made the decision that I was healed from my allergies, took me home, and immediately ceased the strict food rotation I was on. She began feeding me as she would any other child my age. I'll leave you to your own conclusions as to why, but it worked. I was no longer crazy allergic to food anymore.

Growing up, I had a lot of colds and ear infections. I didn't go to public school and wasn't exposed to a lot of people. My mom had a deep fear of anyone who even had a hint of a cold. At her extreme, she would wash everything they had touched after they left the room.

Around the time that I was eleven, my mom, my sister and I were getting a lot of sinus infections. It got to the point that my mom didn't even have to take us to the doctor. She could just call his office, and he would have an antibiotic phoned in for us.

I never thought of myself as having a weight problem until I was twelve years old. I was a very normal, healthy size 6 or 8, weighing about 125 pounds; but I had acquired my mom's bust and also a butt of my own. She was fitting me for an Easter dress she was making for me, when my mom remarked, "Wow, your butt is getting really big."

I hadn't really thought about criticizing my body until that point, and now the damage was done. Instead of tailoring the dress to me and properly fitting it to accommodate my rear, my mom just made the whole thing a size larger. It fit like a shapeless sack.

It was a couple of years after starting the repeated doses of antibiotics that I began feeling depressed. It may have started as difficulty sleeping. I remember the doctor suggesting that I take Benadryl before going to bed as a non-addictive sleep aid. While this helped me sleep, it decreased the rest I got from sleep and increased the difficulty in getting up in the morning. I would be in a fog for most of the day after using Benadryl to sleep.

By the age of fourteen, I was officially diagnosed with depression. I had started harming myself and even had occasional thoughts of suicide. I was unhappy about everything.

Because of my mom's comments, I had started a diet roller coaster. Healthy eating was not something that my mother modeled well. Her idea of breakfast was 1/3 of a mug of coffee with 1/3 of a mug of water and 1/3 of a mug of that really yummy sugary French vanilla creamer. That was consumed with two cake donuts, the kind that comes in the long sleeves in the grocery store.

My mother was also unhappy with her own weight. For support, she was willing to let me try all the crazy diets she tried with her. There was the cabbage soup one where you can eat all the cabbage soup you want as well as one other food a day for a week. This one was touted as the one that helped people in hospitals lose 10 pounds in seven days.

Well, I couldn't choke down the cabbage soup. And the other food item you were allowed to eat was also equally unappetizing for a fourteen-year-old such as raw, plain tomato slices. I think I lasted about three days of eating almost nothing until I broke when my dad and sister stopped for Taco Bell, which is still my absolute favorite fast food.

Another failed crash diet was an attempt at Atkins. I didn't really understand what exactly I was allowed to eat and again felt like I was starving. That lasted for three or four days when I gave in to pancakes on a Saturday morning.

My best friend and I would try to see who could go the longest without eating or who could eat the least amount of calories for multiple days in a row. None of this ever lead to any weight loss, and I continued to beat myself up for my lack of control as the weight continued to inch up.

The inability to control my weight contributed to the depression. I was desperate to feel good about myself and thought that being skinny would help me accomplish that. Because I didn't have the self-control, as I told myself in my brain, to be anorexic, and I was unable to make myself puke, I purchased some ipecac syrup to assist myself in being bulimic. Thank the Lord that only lasted for one night.

After needing antidepressants for most of a year, the family doctor told me I would need them for the rest of my life. At the age of fifteen, this was a huge emotional blow. I saw what happened to depressed people as they got older by watching my mother. She couldn't control her weight on or off antidepressants. And I never saw her feeling anything other than miserable for more than a day or two at a time.

When I was sixteen on the day I was to begin taking piano lessons, which I was very much looking forward to, I had my first migraine headache. I spent the day in bed but still managed to make it to my lesson because I wanted to go so badly.

After that, I started getting tension headaches most days. I had chiropractic adjustments, prescription muscle relaxers, nothing helped. I'm sure my mother gave me some of her Vicodin more than once. But I preferred the pain to the foggy, knocked out feeling of the prescriptions.

In addition to all of this, it became increasingly more difficult to get out of bed in the mornings. I never felt rested. Some of the antidepressants the family doctor tried putting me on would keep me awake and leave me feeling bugged out.

I had really bad hormonal imbalances which left me with extremely heavy periods. They were accompanied by about five days of awful PMS and a few days of painful cramping. My parents never offered to get me birth control, and I never asked for it, partly because I didn't know it could provide symptom relief. I'm grateful now that I didn't start on it at such an early age.

I thought a lot of my depression and tension headaches would go away when I moved out. Living with my mother was a constant state of fear. At any moment she could swing from one extreme to another. She was quite often physically and verbally abusive.

Still, it took me some time to work up the courage to fully move out. I was afraid of the repercussions and her anger. I was twenty when I finally moved out, thanks to my then-boyfriend now-husband Daniel. He encouraged me to see that no one should have to live in the conditions of being around my mother.

That year, while I was dating him, I turned 21 and began an almost yearly battle with strep throat. For the next several years, like clockwork, right around my birthday, I would get knocked down for almost a week with strep.

It was a month or two before we got married that I started trying to figure out the birth control thing. That began years of an emotional roller coaster with breakthrough bleeding nearly every single day. Then, I finally had some relief from the bleeding when I got an IUD put in.

While I no longer was bleeding as often, I didn't realize the mood swings and other issues it was causing. It wasn't until I got the first one taken out and the second one put in did my husband and I realize that it made me really emotionally unstable and contributed to me getting a yeast infection after my period each month.

My depression and pain levels kept increasing as my energy levels decreased. Some days felt like my head and shoulders were in a vise. I had watched my mom live half her life in bed because of depression and pain issues. I struggled with wanting to live if it meant that I was going to live like that. Quite often, I dealt with panic attacks, too.

My husband and I did begin to start figuring out the weight issues. We were both our heaviest ever when we got married and after about seven years of effort, we managed to lose a combined 130 pounds.

In spite of my pain and fatigue, we both really enjoyed running and began training for running events. I wanted to help others lose weight now that we had succeeded, and we both ended up becoming personal trainers and opening our own fitness studio. I wanted others with chronic pain to realize that they should still workout. Running and leading Zumba classes contributed to a positive mood for me. And no matter how much I did or didn't work out, I was going to hurt anyway. I figured I might as well feel better emotionally if I was going to be in pain anyway.

In an attempt to find something to help with the pain and depression, I participated in a double-blind clinical study for Cymbalta. The research was to see if it would benefit people with Fibromyalgia. While I had never been formally diagnosed with Fibromyalgia (mostly because I didn't have health insurance and didn't regularly see a doctor), I had the same symptoms that my mother who had been diagnosed suffered from.

While the Cymbalta did help my mood, it didn't allow me to sleep. Not until I was sitting still driving a car that is. Every time I got behind the wheel, I was in danger of passing out. But if I laid down to sleep at night, I was lucky to get three hours of restless sleep.

Once the study was over, we tried to pay for the prescription out of pocket, but we couldn't afford it beyond a month. That was one of the worst withdrawals ever. I wouldn't wish it on an enemy. I was dizzy and moody for months.

We had started our fitness studio and I was working two outside jobs to help support us when my amazing mom-in-law told me about her natural health practitioner, Karen. There was an upcoming class that Karen was holding at her store/office in a city about 25 minutes away. It was very affordable at just $15. I rearranged my multiple schedules to make it work.

Karen's husband Ed called me a couple of hours before the class started explaining that everyone else had been unable to attend the class that evening. Would I be able to reschedule for a different week? I told him that I understood if they needed to cancel the class, but that I wasn't sure with my schedule when I would be able to make it out there. Karen graciously held the class for just me that day.

I know now, looking back, that I probably would not have spoken up and gotten what I needed from that evening if there had been more people there. The class was based on a little booklet that Karen had put together from her years in natural health. The topic was the basics that people need to understand about their bodies in order for them to be healthy. We'll review that information in the next chapter. Because it is so simple, I think that many feel it is unimportant, but it really is necessary for our health.

Karen reached the page in her booklet where she talked about how many bowel movements a day someone should have. As she described it, "Three trains in, three trains out." This is where I held up my hand and said, "Wait a minute. I struggle to have three bowel movements a week. How is three a day possible?"

In her sweet, motherly, no-nonsense tone, Karen replied, "Girl, we gotta get your body moving!"

Karen spent two hours of her time, something that she would normally charge a client $150 for, with just me that evening. After the class, we went out front to her shop and she muscle tested me for an herbal cleanse.

Muscle testing is just a way of asking your body what would make it stronger. We all have an electrical current that runs through us because we are made up of protons, neutrons, and electrons: positive, negative, and neutrally charged particles. Everything in the world has a small electrical current as well because everything has these charged particles. When you introduce a supplement into your electrical field, you can see if it makes you stronger or weaker. That is muscle testing in the simplest nutshell.

Also, when I talk about a cleanse, as I will throughout this book, I'm never talking about a glued to your toilet while water pours from your butt kind of thing. That is not working with your body. I'm talking about something that helps your body removes toxins and wastes in a gentle manner.

Any time that you take a "cleanse" that causes intestinal cramping, abdominal pain, and being glued to the toilet with water coming out your butt, that is not working with your body. A cleanse should not cause a lot of discomforts. And if it isn't helping you produce solid bowel movements, then it is either way too strong for you and you should drastically decrease how much you are taking, or it isn't the right one for you. There are so many cleanses out there. Once you take one that works with your body, you'll wonder why you ever fought through one of the scary ones.

Back to my story now. Karen asked my body, through muscle response testing aka kinesiology, which cleanse would be best for me to start with in order to help me have more bowel movements a day. The cleanse was relatively inexpensive. I think it was $22 retail. But I only had the $15 for the class in my pocket that day.

I promised to come back in the next couple of weeks for the cleanse, but Karen understood how severe my situation was. The Lord must have been working through her that day because she did something out of the ordinary. She sent me home without charging me for the cleanse.

It was difficult for me to accept this. And it's something that I've learned not to do very often. Those of us in the industry of helping people learn the difficult way that people don't appreciate what you give them for free.

I accepted this gift and used it. Overnight, I saw results in my bowel movements and within a day or two, I noticed a drastic difference in my body's energy. It practically doubled overnight.

The bottle lasted me about two weeks during which time I took it faithfully every day. I couldn't believe how much better I felt. But after two weeks, I ran out. My bowel movements returned to my "normal". And my energy level sunk back down. What on earth had gone wrong?

I went back out to Karen's shop and asked her why I felt as I had before. She explained that my body had been functioning poorly for so long, that it was going to take much more than one cleanse to "fix" me.

This is a big block in people's heads when they start working with a natural health practitioner. We are trying to help your body fix what is at the root of the problem and that takes time. The longer you have had the issue, the deeper the roots of it go in your body.

I continued on with another of the same cleanse, but I also agreed to come out and take more classes from her. This little bottle of liquid herbs was doing for me what no prescription had been able to do. I was finally feeling better. A lot of my mental fog was gone. With the increased energy came a little decrease in my pain levels. I wanted to know more about this natural "magic".

After a couple more classes, I knew that this was what I wanted to do with my life: help others achieve the health possible for them naturally. Working with my body instead of against it made so much sense to me. Taking the plants that God gave us that people have been using successfully for thousands of years and helping others is such a joy and an honor.

I wasn't magically better even after the second bottle of cleanse. There was still a long journey ahead of me to reduce my depression and pain issues. Along the way, I learned that most of the nutrition classes I have taken for my personal training certifications were pretty much useless nonsense.

Initially, I fell into the trap that most people do when they start studying natural health or looking for natural ways to help with specific issues: we look for something that will help the symptom we are dealing with. This is, in essence, trying to use natural medicine the way we use Western medicine: if you have this symptom, then you take this specific thing to help that.

This approach definitely limits the effectiveness of the plants and herbs. I help my clients with symptom relief as we address the root of the issue. But addressing the root is always the best way for long-term health.

For example, I found this certain supplement that was super effective in helping me manage my mood. It contained a jet black cocoa powder. Yes, real chocolate really is magical for your mood! And this stuff worked like a charm. Until it was discontinued. I stock-piled as many boxes of it as I could when I found out it was no longer going to be available. But what was I going to do when my stash ran out?

It took me about five years of studying a naturopathic doctor program to learn how to address the root of my depression instead of just the symptoms. Learning how to do that is where the real ticket to freedom lies. Because once you address the root, then it doesn't matter how many different styles of crutches and bandages are produced. Different products can come and go, and you aren't at the mercy of wondering how to get that specific one that worked for you.

Address the root and the symptoms go away.

I've continued to learn over the years. Learning is a passion of mine. And I want to bring the bigger picture to those of you who are ready to see it. Looking for natural remedies for symptoms is like looking at the backside of just one piece of the puzzle. I hope this book begins to bring some color and clarity of the health puzzle to you and help you realize just how much control you have over how you feel.

The helpless and hopeless feelings you have about changing your health are just because you bought a lie that it is outside of you to change it. I believed that lie for so long as well. Believing that lie can make you suicidal. I definitely was at times. Because if life was just miserable days of existing in pain and feeling tiredness so deep that no amount of sleep can fix it, then I didn't want to do it anymore. Helping my clients see through that lie is the most important first step I help them with.

My first meeting with Karen was the beginning of that fog lifting from my life. I hope that this book can begin to lift the fog for you to see what is possible.

Losing weight the easy way.

As I mentioned before, I've done a lot of diets in my life. My earliest attempts were no healthier than starvation.

When I met my husband Daniel, he had spent most of his life overweight. His mom and sister were a healthy weight while Daniel and his dad were overweight. Growing up, Daniel just assumed that was the way things were: you were either a healthy weight or overweight and you couldn't do anything about it.

As a young adult, Daniel had also tried a lot of fad diets, but none of them were any more helpful than a yo-yo. When we met, we were both ready for something better.

We originally tried a mainstream weight loss plan that involved counting points. Well, I'm too good at math for my own good sometimes. After several months of doing that, I had figured out how to maximize how much food we could eat for the fewest amount of points, and eventually, we plateaued.

Then we went the more tedious method of counting calories. If you have ever counted calories, you know how much time that requires day after day unless you want to eat the same exact thing every single day which gets boring and isn't very healthy.

We've definitely gone up and down with our weight over the years, only able to lose weight and keep it off when we count calories. We did lose a combined 130 pounds doing this, which is nothing to scoff about. But both of us did end up regaining our weight.

Then, when I started studying natural health, I learned about healthy ways of reducing calories such as fasts. My first fast was a five-day juice fast. I had never had so much energy in my life. I always feel amazing when I juice fast, unlike some of the other people I have taken through a five-day juice fast.

Most of the weight loss on a five day fast of any sort is water weight. Part of this is because your body is able to reduce its internal inflammation on a fast. Our body holds onto the water as a buffer against inflammation. The parts of your body that are inflamed swell: your body is concentrating fluids there as a buffer.

When we fast, our body can work on cleaning things out. As inflammation decreases, the need for extra fluids in the body decreases. Hence, we lose water weight.

Fasting is a great jumping board for improving health. But any time that we return to the way we did things before, our body and our circumstances will return to what they were before. When we stop taking care of anything, it returns to chaos.

Think about your kitchen counters. If you don't clean them for a week, what happens? They get dirty, right? Can you just clean them once and be done with it? No. We have to create daily habits of cleaning in order to have clean counters.

This is the way it is in the body. If there is something that your body needs help cleaning out, it can't just be a one and done situation. We need to do it on a regular basis in order to maintain it.

When I was a personal trainer, I would train a lot of clients who wanted to lose weight. I could often get them great results; but, as soon as they quit working with me, they would eventually return to how they were before. Losing weight is a form of cleaning out your body; and it requires maintenance the same as anything else we want to keep orderly in our lives: a garden, a clean vehicle, a clean house. It requires action by somebody to keep things neat and clean.

If we have a messy house, and we don't want it to be that way, then we have to clean it on a regular basis. In the same way, if we have an overweight body, then we need to make changes that we can maintain. If we have health symptoms, we have to work to restore and maintain health.

From my experience of working with people who want to lose weight through the years, those who are doing it just to lose weight never keep it off. I've seen a 95% fail rate there.

However, the most success I have ever had of keeping weight off is when I focus on taking care of my body, of being the healthiest that I can be. When I change my focus from my weight to my health, the weight takes care of itself.

There is a little known fact that stops even people who count calories every single day and never break their diet from maintaining their weight loss. The body stores toxins that it cannot process in our fat cells. When the body runs out of storage area, it can create more of these little toxin storage units called fat cells.

When we lose fat, our body releases those toxins and they begin circulating again. This is why you may feel worse or even flu-like when you lose weight or go on a fast as your body is releasing more toxins than it can deal with.

Yes, our liver is responsible for processing those toxins for removal, but every body part requires nutrients to run properly, something most of us are starving for. If the liver is missing one of those nutrients, then it can't do its work, and the toxins pile up.

This begins the yo-yo weight loss cycle. The body has toxins it can't deal with so it begins to store them in the fat cells. We get unhappy with our weight and go on a "diet". As we lose fat, the toxins begin circulating again. At a certain point, our body won't allow anymore fat to be lost because it can't handle the toxin overload. That is when we plateau and eventually regain our weight.

What I lead my clients through is a process that helps the body over the course of several years, if necessary, process the toxins it has been storing and balance the microbiome, which we haven't even talked about yet in this book, in order to maintain a healthy weight easily.

Keep reading to get an overview of that process.

Key Learnings

Crash and fad diets don't contribute to long-term changes

Frequent antibiotic use contributes to bigger health issues.

Exercise contributes to a positive mood.

We can ask our body what nutrients it needs through muscle response testing.

Cleansing should be gentle and work with your body.

We can't repair our health in one month.

Always seek to address the root of the health problem.

Only YOU have the ability to repair your health.

Focusing on health is a long-term solution for weight loss.

Our health and our bodies require regular maintenance.

Toxins that our body can't process are stored in fat and contribute to extra weight.

Write down anything else from this chapter that you want to remember.

7

Basics of Health

This chapter is based upon bullet points I pulled from the pamphlet Karen took me through in my very first class with her. I include this information here because even the greatest researchers among my clients didn't know all of these basics. I have had to review them with every single person I have worked with. These are foundational for improving your health no matter how good or bad it is right now.

Natural Health is Preventative

Have you ever gone to a doctor when you were healthy? Have you ever gone to a chiropractor when something didn't hurt? Have you ever walked into a health store and said, "I feel great. I have no symptoms. I sleep like a log. Nothing in my body hurts. What do I need to do to maintain this?"

If you are like just about everyone else in the United States, you probably haven't. We aren't taught to maintain anything that is going well. We are taught to be reactive. If it isn't broken, don't fix it.

The original wooden wheel wasn't broken, but someone thought it could be better. Candles made out of wax and cotton provided light, but someone decided that a light bulb could be better. The rotary dial telephones attached to our walls thirty years ago allowed us to call a loved one across the country or across the world just fine, but aren't the new cell phones we carry much nicer?

The idea of "this is good, but how could it be better?" is how natural health shines the brightest. Remember how I said a few pages ago that the Chinese only pay their doctor for as long as they remain healthy? It is easier to keep someone in good health than it is to help someone regain good health.

The more proactive we are, the easier it will be. The higher the standards we have for our health, the easier it will be to maintain. The more we ask, "This is good, but how could it be even better?" the happier we will be.

Key Learnings

When we ask how we can make something better, we can always find a way for it to improve, even with our health.

What direction is your health heading?

In the five years that I worked behind a retail health store counter, I heard so many people talk about the health issues that don't bother them enough to do something about it.

"I'm not sleeping well, but it's not bothering me enough that I want to take something for it."

"It hurts to do things that I love to do, but that isn't enough for me to want to spend money on it."

Those are just a couple of examples of what I heard nearly every day for years. If your body is in a declining state, do you believe that it will either get better on its own or continue to get worse? Does your house ever clean itself? Does your garden ever weed itself? Why do you think you can ignore your health and it will eventually get better?

If you continue to do the same things you are doing now, and eat the same way, and live the same way, and take the same drugstore supplements, your health will continue to progress in the direction it has been. Is that the direction you want to go in?

If your health continues in that direction, where will you be in one year? In five years? In ten? Is that what you want for your life?

If not, it is time to course correct now.

Key Learning

If you continue the habits and patterns that are creating your current health, your health will continue in the direction it is going.

Germ Theory vs Terrain Theory

At the time of this writing, my husband and I have owned a gym for almost eight years. At the entrance, there is a wall dispenser of hand sanitizing gel.

A certain client of his was always deathly afraid of germs and getting sick. Whenever she would come to work out, and she often had her child in tow, she would slather them both in the sanitizing gel. While she didn't get sick any more than most of the people we worked with, her child was always sick.

I see a lot of people focus on buying antibacterial soaps at the store. For many people, that is the only stipulation they have about the hand soap they buy.

We've all seen the commercials for these soaps: "Proven to kill 99.9% of germs on contact." But is that really helping us to not get sick? Even the FDA doesn't think so anymore. I found this article on their website titled "Antibacterial Soap? You can skip it. Use Plain Soap and Water". It was current as of 5/16/19:

In essence, they come right out and say that the benefits of these soaps aren't any better than regular soap and water. We've been using these soaps for long enough that their antibacterial ingredient, triclosan, might be more dangerous to our health and the environment than we've thought before.

The FDA says the information doesn't apply to antibacterial sanitizing gels and sprays, but I still recommend using them sparingly.

The microbiome is a much bigger organism than you might imagine. For those of you who are new to the term, it's the name for the trillions of microbes that live in us and on us. In fact, these good and bad bugs that call us home outnumber our own human cells ten to one.

Let's think of these little guys as foot soldiers for a minute. A healthy microbiome, which translates to a healthier human, should be comprised of about 80% good foot soldiers. We can't ever get rid of all the bad guys, and it isn't necessary as long as we maintain a good majority over them.

The problem that a lot of people are experiencing is having the opposite ratio of good guys to bad guys. They only have 20 trillion foot soldiers fighting for them and 80 trillion soldiers fighting against them and their health.

How does this imbalance happen? When we routinely bomb all the soldiers, good and bad alike, with antibiotics and combine that with the Standard American Diet (SAD) that only feeds the bad guys our entire microbiome is effectively destroyed. Can you imagine a country ever winning a war by only feeding the enemy troops?

The enemy troops in us love and thrive off of things that are unhealthy for us: chemicals, medications, heavy metals, yeast by-products (yeasts in the gut like candida), junk foods, processed foods, etc.

Every time we consume something by eating, drinking, touching it, or breathing it in, we are feeding and supporting our good bugs or the bad bugs. Which would you like to support? It's your choice.

Studies have shown that a poor microbiome contributes to obesity, type two diabetes, insulin resistance, and other metabolic diseases. A large issue is having too many Firmicutes and too little Bacteroidetes. The ratio of these two bacteria can have a direct effect on whether or not you can maintain a healthy weight.

You can find more information here:
https://www.ncbi.nlm.nih.gov/pmc/articles/PMC3705322/

Have you ever experienced the inability to lose weight no matter how much you diet and exercise? If your microbiome isn't conducive to you being skinny, then your weight loss plans are doomed from the start.

I have seen pictures of identical twins, both human and animal, where one was skinny and the other grossly overweight. They are able to induce this with lab rats. What is the difference? Their microbiome. When one has a healthy microbiome, they are able to maintain a healthy weight naturally and easily

Identical twins start out genetically the same. Through diet and lifestyle choices, their microbiome will change to reflect their habits.

Are you ready for the good news? We can undo the damage and restore the proper ratio of good guys versus bad guys in our bodies. However, the process takes time. If you have been feeding and cultivating the bad guys for 20 years, you can't change the ratio to what it should be overnight.

This is all about establishing long-term habits and patterns that support overall health. I always encourage people to think about their microbiome as a garden. If your garden is full of weeds, it takes some time to clear them out and plant new seeds and see the fruit from those seeds.

The fruit of a healthy microbiome is a healthy human.

We need to think of this journey as a marathon, not a sprint. We can sprint to buy healthy groceries for the week, but we can't grow a fruit-producing fruit tree overnight.

I have friends who have walked a marathon in eight hours. I have run one in four and a half. I have been at events where the winner finished in one hour, forty-five minutes. We can all take it at our own pace. We are only competing against ourselves here.

However, a marathon has a beginning and an ending, and this marathon is our life. If you have been off the course for a while now, the sooner you decide to get back on, no matter what pace you are going, the sooner you can start to make progress.

Key Learnings

Antibacterial soaps kill both good and bad bacteria.

A healthy microbiome is comprised of 80% good bacteria to 20% bad.

Our habits and lifestyle determine whether we are supporting our good bacteria or the bad.

Cultivating a healthy microbiome will help you manage your weight.

We need to think about creating healthy habits for life, not just for a week.

Write down the key points from this chapter that you would like to remember.

Healthy Plants and Animals

Have you ever seen two people grow similar plants in their garden on adjacent properties? One person's plants flourished and looked beautiful without the need for herbicides or pesticides while their neighbor's plants struggled and were being consumed by pests.

What is the difference? They both are being exposed to the same "bugs". The difference is the soil. This is where terrain theory comes in.

We can't get away from bugs as much as we try. But just like plants, the healthier we are, the less pest-resistant we are.

Organic farmers know the importance of properly balancing their soil for healthier plants. How do they make the soil healthier? By correcting it's acid/alkaline balance and adding nutrients.

In the same way, when we balance our bodies, we become disease and pest resistant. Not only can our immune system fight them off better, but we become undesirable to them as well.

The Importance of Minerals

What happens to your body when it dies? It decomposes and eventually becomes soil. What do plants need that soil provides? Minerals.

Plants cannot flourish without minerals. Animals eat plants and obtain their minerals that way. Our bodies can't function normally without minerals.

I'll probably say this multiple times throughout this book because it's an important concept: diseases have two causes. If you have a disease, you either have a nutrient deficiency, some sort of toxicity in the body, or a combination of the two..

A deficiency in the body can also be a cause of toxicity. If we are deficient in good bacteria, then bad bacteria flourishes.

I already said that the liver requires nutrients in order to function as the body's filter. These include iron, oxygen, calcium (in an organic form), vitamin A, and iodine to name just the top 5. If the liver can't process toxins, then they remain in the body. If the colon doesn't get enough water and fiber, then it can't eliminate toxins properly.

All of these actions require nutrients. We all know the importance of vitamins. B-vitamins and d3 are common vitamins that we all know we need. Without minerals, vitamins can do nothing in the body. Minerals are the main building block of the body.

We need all of them for proper body function. The best way to get a wide variety of minerals into your body is to consume herbs from a reputable company. For an example of a basic, customizable supplement protocol that I would recommend for anyone, as well as a link to the supplements I recommend for my clients, check out the book bonuses area: BookBonuses.NHWarriors.com.

Key Learning

Life requires minerals

Digestion

Digestion determines whether what you are eating becomes a toxin to your body or something you can use. If your body can't properly digest your food, then it ferments and spoils in your body, and you can't get the nutrients from it.

The vast majority of digestion issues are from either an insufficiency in stomach acid or a deficiency of enzymes.

When we experience heartburn or reflux, we immediately assume that we have too much stomach acid. The reverse is usually the case, especially in adults over the age of thirty. I am beginning to see the hydrochloric acid deficiency more often even in adults younger than thirty now as our digestive system's ability is declining at younger and younger ages. To correct this, we need to focus on ways to increase stomach acid instead of decreasing it as conventional medicine tells us.

One of the most harmful toxins that arise from poor digestion is undigested proteins. Protein requires a highly acidic environment in the stomach in order to be broken down.

The symptoms of poor digestion are numerous. You may experience reflux or heartburn, gas or bloating after meals. The stomach may feel like it is slow to empty after meals or food sits heavy in the stomach. Intestinal issues such as candida or an overgrowth of small intestinal bacteria can flourish. Ultimately, this can all lead to constipation, diarrhea, or an alternation between the two.

A lack of enzymes can also lead to food not being broken down properly. A deficiency of enzymes is caused by not consuming enough living, raw food in the diet and too much dead food (cooked or processed). Fresh fruits and vegetables contain the enzymes needed to digest them.

Enzymes are catalysts that help certain processes happen. There are processes the body completes in seconds that wouldn't be able to happen over the course of a million years without the necessary enzymes. Enzymes are required for life.

Fresh fruits and vegetables rot because of the enzymes they contain. All enzymes are destroyed by the time any food is heated to 130 degrees Fahrenheit, which would make for a very unsatisfactory bowl of soup. Any time we cook food, we destroy the enzymes.

We are born with a limited supply of enzymes. The more cooked, canned, and processed food we eat, the more we use up our enzyme supply. This is why my client's health improves very quickly when we start adding enzymes to their daily program.

Enzymes are very different from probiotics. Many people that I talked to in my retail store are unaware of the difference. Probiotics are the good bacteria that we need to populate our intestines. The word means "for (pro) life (bio)". They are a very necessary part of our immune system.

Enzymes break down the food we eat for proper digestion and nutrient absorption.

Our supply of enzymes and our body's ability to break down food properly can influence the health of these good bacteria.

Key Learning

Digestive difficulties start with either too little stomach acid, not enough enzymes, or both.

Enzymes are required for life.

We deplete our enzyme stores by eating too much dead food and not enough living food.

Enzymes are destroyed when heated.

Enzymes are catalysts: they help things happen as a rate fast enough to sustain life.

Probiotics are good bacteria.

Write down any other points you would like to remember.

Intestines and Antibiotics

The very word antibiotic means "against (anti) life (bio)". Antibiotics are indiscriminate: they attack and kill all bacteria in the body that they come into contact with: the good with the bad.

A good way of thinking about the care that our intestinal flora (microbiome) needs is to think about a lush green lawn. People who have thick luscious green lawns that make you want to take off your shoes and run barefoot through it have worked hard on their lawns.

A healthy lawn requires regular feeding, watering, and weeding. Roundup, a popular glyphosate based herbicide, affects a lawn the same way antibiotics affect our internal bacteria, killing the good and the bad. If you spray Roundup on a lawn and then leave it, what happens? Everything dies; the weeds take over. If you don't replant grass and care for it, weeds always take over.

This is the same for our internal microbiome. If we take an antibiotic, it wipes out the whole thing. And if we don't seek to replant the good bacteria, then the bad are able to take over. This is why women are prone to yeast infections after a round of antibiotics. The bad was allowed to flourish because there were no good bugs in there to keep them in check.

A yeast infection is the least of the issues caused though. By the time that yeast can affect us externally, it has been proliferating on the inside. Our external body is merely a reflection of the internal conditions of the body. Athlete's foot, psoriasis, eczema, acne, rosacea, and other similar skin conditions all reflect an unhealthy internal microbiome.

Key Learning

Antibiotics kill both good and bad bacteria.

If we have an external skin condition, it is a reflection of the state of our internal microbiome.

Four Organs of Elimination

Our body has four main organs or systems responsible for eliminating the waste: the skin, kidneys, colon, and lungs.

The Skin

The skin is our largest organ of elimination. Any unwanted skin condition is a sign that the other elimination pathways are not open and working optimally, and that a large amount of the workload is falling back on the skin. Dry skin brushing is a really helpful way to assist the skin in eliminating by removing dead cells and stimulating the flow of the lymphatic system, which is key in eliminating body waste.

Using a natural bristle brush, brush your skin while it is dry before you shower. Using long strokes, start at the bottom of your feet and brush up and towards the heart. A good sign that your skin needs help detoxing is if you don't sweat when you workout.

This used to be my experience: I would go for a run or lead a Zumba Fitness class and would barely sweat until I started dry brushing my skin.

The Kidneys

Our kidneys eliminate wastes and help to control the pH balance of the body by eliminating through the bladder. Most of the cellular wastes removed by the body are eliminated through the kidneys. Urine should be almost colorless and odorless unless you have recently taken a vitamin B-complex. This will temporarily turn your urine bright yellow. This is not unwanted and is a sign that your body actually processed the vitamins.

There are very few people I have met who drink enough water. A good rule of thumb is to drink half of your body weight in ounces a day as a bare minimum. This would mean that a 160-pound person should drink at least 80 ounces of water a day. There are occasions when we should drink more than that amount such as if it is an exceptionally warm day, if you are doing physical activity, or if you are experiencing congestion.

Adding some fresh lemon juice to warm, not hot, water and drinking it first thing in the morning helps balance body pH from acids that accumulate overnight. Citrus fruits have an alkalizing effect on the body. Proper urine pH is 6.4.

The Colon

It is amazing the number of people who only have one bowel movement per day or less. This is not proper elimination. Also, when you think about the quantity of food consumed compared to the amount of poop coming out you can see another disparity.

My husband had a personal training client who started working with him for the goal of weight loss. He had her counting calories and working out four or five hours a week. But she was only having one or two bowel movements a week. She thought her body was running so efficiently on the quantity of food she was eating that she didn't need to have more frequent bowel movements than that. Not having regular bowel movements will definitely keep the scale stuck.

Even on a juice fast or during other periods of time when we aren't consuming solid foods, we should still be having solid bowel movements. During these times, it may only be once a day. Half of the stool we pass is waste from the good bacteria in our intestines. If we have very little stool we are passing, that may be because we don't have enough good bacteria.

Normal bowel movements, as a rule, should be solid in consistency while not being too hard or difficult to pass. They should be a medium brown in color, should not have a strong smell, should sink, and should be a decent size around. If we laid it out end on end, the total amount of stool we pass each day should equal at least the length of our arm. Any deviations from that normal are a sign that there are malfunctions in the body that need to be addressed.

Some of the best things to do for a healthy colon is to eat plenty of raw fruits and vegetables. These provide the fiber which is food for our good bacteria. Also, it's important to supplement with probiotics.

I know I'm going to sound insane when I say this, but enemas are a regular part of my colon care. The use of water in the colon for health and cleansing purposes dates back thousands of years. If you take the time to research how to do one properly, they are very safe. One of the most common errors made with enemas are from using liquid that is too hot. I typically temp my liquids and make sure they are no hotter than 100 degrees Fahrenheit.

Start with a very small amount of fluid and work your way up to a quart or two at a time. And make your own enema solutions from quality ingredients rather than buying one at the store.

One client of mine thought that I was crazy for suggesting enemas. Once she noticed how much energy she had after she did a coffee enema, she began enjoying them as well.

When I have a cold or any kind of respiratory congestion, the first thing I make time for is a series of enemas. Congestion in the body correlates to too much congestion in the intestinal tract. Enemas can do wonders for clearing up congested sinuses and allowing someone to breathe freely again. Also, I find that I get over colds much faster than my husband when I utilize enemas and he does not.

The Lungs

When Rebekah first talked to me at my retail health store, she asked me what she could do for her child's asthma. She thought I was crazy when I said that it was caused by a poorly functioning intestinal system and an imbalanced microbiome. So many issues in our body go back to whether or not the intestinal and digestive systems are functioning properly and whether the microbiome is healthy. After working with me for about four months on her own health issues and applying what she was doing for her daughter, the child no longer needed asthma medication. Addressing the gut was key. It has now been well over a year since her daughter has needed asthma medication. (Dec. 2019)

The lungs contribute to the pH balance in our body as well. When we exhale, we breathe out acid waste. Regular exercise is very important for the lungs.

Key Learning

Our body has four primary organs responsible for eliminating wastes: the skin, kidneys, colon, and lungs.

The skin is our largest organ of elimination. We can support it through dry skin brushing.

We can support our kidneys by drinking enough water. A good rule of thumb is to drink half your body weight in ounces of water each day.

For every meal we eat, we should have a solid bowel movement.

Enemas are helpful for clearing congestion anywhere in the body.

Regular exercise is helpful for supporting the lungs.

Write down any other points you would like to remember from this chapter.

Two causes of disease

The two causes of disease are nutritional deficiency and toxicity. It's really that easy. When people start working with me, they often want to discuss their medical diagnoses and all the tests and lab work they have had done. I don't need to know what disease someone has in order to help them. I can ask them questions about what symptoms they are experiencing in order to address possible deficiencies or toxicities.

When we look back at the earliest symptoms someone experienced on the long road to a medical diagnosis, we can see which body system was the first domino to fall in a long chain that inevitably leads to a disease.

By correcting the deficiencies and toxicities that cause those symptoms, we can begin to help the body restore health by addressing that first domino that fell. Often, the disease is six or ten or even more "dominoes" down the line. We can't get the part of the body back on line without righting the ones on top of it first.

When you can wrap your mind around this concept of two causes, you can become empowered to take control of your health. The whole idea of natural health is self-empowerment. You have the ultimate control over whether your body is diseased or healthy.

There are five physical factors that contribute to these two causes. We can break down the two causes of disease by looking at the five factors that contribute to them.

Deficiency

Nutritional deficiencies can occur when someone is eating a poor diet such as too many processed and devitalized foods in ratio to fresh, living food and, also, when digestion is poor.

The food supply in the United States is mostly dead and devitalized. This is why we have such a need for quality health supplements. Our modern farming practices don't support the growth of produce that contains high mineral content.

My mom-in-law and nephew just got back from a mission trip to Uganda. They showed pictures of a farm field there. They don't just farm one crop for acres and acres. Instead, many crops are interspersed. This preserves the nutrients in the soil and makes the crops much more healthy.

The native Americans didn't farm fields of just one crop either. As an example, they have a trio known as the three sisters that were commonly planted together: corn, beans, and squash. The corn provides a structure for the beans to climb, and the squash keeps the surrounding soil relatively free of weeds with their broad leaves. Each plant works in harmony to acquire different nutrients from the soil and contributes other nutrients back to the soil.

Modern farming practices leave the soil and, subsequently, our food devoid of nutrients and require massive amounts of pesticides and herbicides.

Ancient cultures have been using supplements for millennia. It is only recently that we have the benefit of being able to take herbs internally in the form of a handy little capsule. Traditional Chinese medicine and Ayurvedic medicine would require people to drink bitter-tasting herbs in the form of tea. Sometimes several cups of this would be called for each day. Consider that the next time you complain about having to swallow a handful of pills. If you would rather, you can open your herbal capsules and make a tea with them, but I doubt that you will always find it very palatable.

Toxins

As much as we try, we can't steer clear of toxins. They exist in the air we breathe, surfaces we touch, the food we eat, and the water we drink. They include such things as chemicals, pesticides, herbicides, chlorine, fluorine, parasites, heavy metals, EMF exposure, bacteria, and viruses.

Toxins get in the way of normal body function. Some of them resemble key nutrients we need and will fill receptor cells in the body blocking the essential nutrients from filling its proper place. As an example, much of our drinking water has fluoride and chlorine added to it. These chemicals block the receptor (receiving) sites in the body for iodine, a necessary nutrient for thyroid and liver health.

Living toxins such as viruses, bacteria, and yeasts can create waste in the body that needs to be eliminated. There is no end to the damage they can do if we don't assist the body in keeping their numbers low.

Toxin overload can be associated with a deficiency as mentioned early. If our organs of elimination don't have the nutrients they need to function as they were designed, they can't break down and safely eliminate toxins.

Stress and Accidents

Stress contributes to disease because it contributes to both deficiency and toxicity. During times of stress, we use up a lot more nutrients than normal, especially magnesium and b-vitamins. Most of us don't compensate for this during times of stress by taking three to four times more of the vital nutrients our body is burning through. We then wonder why we feel so run down.

Not having these nutrients contributes to symptoms such as an inability to handle stressors, depression, anxiety, high blood pressure, poor cognition, and more.

Stress also produces toxins in the body. In the same way that happy moods produce dopamine, serotonin, and other endorphins, poor moods produce harmful hormones. Stress also weakens our immune system and allows viruses, bacteria, and fungi to proliferate.

Many of my clients can trace the beginning of their health problems back to a major stressor such as an abusive situation, accident, surgery, an antibiotic, a long period of working at a job that made them unhappy, and other similar situations.

We can help the body deal with stress in a healthy way. The category of herbs called adaptogens is really beneficial for adapting and dealing with stress in a healthy way. Just be sure to take enough from a high-quality brand.

Some of my favorite adaptogens that can be found in blends together include ashwagandha, astragalus, eleuthero, rhodiola, schisandra, and suma.

You can find links to some of my favorite blends in your bonus area: BookBonuses.NHWarriors.com

Drugs

Drugs, whether recreational or prescription, can contribute to a deficiency or toxicity in the body. Many prescriptions have a harmful effect on our microbiome, killing our good bacteria. Others deplete the body of essential vitamins and minerals or stop our body's elimination channels.

Recreational drugs can take the place of receptor sites in the body. Smoking depletes the body of vitamin c while the nicotine can block niacin (b3) receptor sites in the body. That is just one example of many.

Two of the most socially acceptable drugs are caffeine and sugar, both of which can have harmful effects on the body.

Key Learnings

Diseases are caused by toxicity, deficiencies, or a combination of the two.

We need to focus on the earliest symptoms we experienced when trying to heal from disease.

Herbs can be taken in tea or capsule form.

Modern farming practices don't support produce with healthy mineral supplies.

Toxins get in the way of normal body function.

Stress can cause both deficiencies and toxicity.

Drugs and chemicals can block important receptor sites in the body.

Write down any other points from this chapter that you would like to remember.

Some Basic Body Needs

Our body requires fresh air, not stale indoor air or polluted city air.

We need sunshine on a nearly daily basis. Getting sunlight on our skin is a much more valuable form of acquiring vitamin d than taking a supplement. However, when you live at or above the 45th parallel on the globe, it is impossible to obtain enough vitamin D from the sun.

Water

So many health issues would go away if people were willing to drink enough water.

A long-term customer at my store asked what I suggested for low back pain and kidney irritation.

"How much water are you drinking?" I ask.

"I drink a lot of water," he replies.

"Not enough," his wife blurts out at the same time.

This is not the first time I've suggested that he drink more water. If someone isn't willing to do what is suggested to improve an issue, then I have to assume it isn't bothering them enough to do something about it.

A retired dentist is also a frequent customer at my store. One day he came in asking what to do about his tongue. It was raw, red, swollen, and dry.

"How much water do you drink?" I ask.

"Well that's a good question," he responds. We talk over how a lack of water could be contributing to his issue, and he admits that he doesn't drink a lot of water.

My husband had a personal training client who experienced a lot of headaches, including migraines, and other frequent health conditions. He encouraged her, as he does with all his clients, to drink enough water. She admitted that she never drank water and didn't care for it.

She trained with him for many years. Several years later, when she was no longer a client, we saw her and she happened to mention that her doctor had demanded that she drink more water. Many of the issues and headaches she was dealing with cleared up.

I want to encourage you not to dismiss the most basic information in this book because that is most often where people are lacking and problems can start. This is where people who try to research their diseases fall short. They fail to learn about the basic needs of the body and how all the body systems work together.

We've all heard that we need to drink a lot of water, but do you?

Our Body is Made of Water

Did you know that your body operates on electricity? Every cell in your body has its own mild current. When we examine atoms, we see that they are made of electrically charged particles. Every atom contains these protons, neutrons, and electrons, and every physical thing on our earth is made of atoms.

A hydrated body should be close to 70% water. Water is a good conductor of electricity. Our body's electricity can't work correctly if we aren't hydrated enough.

Difficulty concentrating and thinking? Drink some more water. Nerve pulses in the brain are electrical and require proper hydration. Even very mild dehydration can result in a decrease in cognition. By the time you feel thirsty, you are already dehydrated.

As we age, our sense of thirst dulls. I know a grandmother who has frequently been in the emergency room for bladder and kidney infections because of a lack of water. Her family ended up putting little signs around her apartment saying, "Drink more water" and setting out glasses of water for her to consume each day.

Have you ever found yourself in the kitchen wondering what you want to eat but nothing looks good? We can easily mistake thirst for hunger. Try drinking a glass of water and giving it twenty minutes before going back and looking for a healthy snack. You may find you don't require one at all.

Common knowledge says that a person can live for forty days without food, but we can only live for three to five days without water. If you only put one thing in your mouth today, make it water. It's more important than food.

What does water do for us?

Water is involved in nearly every bodily function including digestion, absorbing nutrients, circulation, excretion, as a transporter of nutrients, building healthy body cells, regulating temperature, and carrying out wastes.

We need to replace the water in our bodies daily. We use up to a pint a day just from breathing. We also lose water through our skin when we sweat and exercise and when we urinate.

Water is needed for your heart

The American Heart Association says hydration is critical for our heart health. Low body water equals low blood volume. When we are dehydrated, our blood is thicker and more difficult to pump. Not enough blood may get to the brain in these cases.

How dehydration happens

We aren't taught as we grow up to pay attention to our bodies. Our body has the ability to let us know what it needs if we would only listen.

Many of us end up mistaking hunger for thirst. And very few people make drinking water a daily habit with reminders if needed.

Symptoms drinking water can help

If my husband or I ever have a headache, which is really infrequent, the first question we ask the other is, "Have you been drinking enough water?" A lot of headaches can be caused by dehydration.

Drinking water also helps bowel and bladder problems. When we don't drink enough water, wastes accumulate in the kidneys and aren't flushed out. These wastes are usually acidic and very irritating to sensitive body tissues.

Some cases of constipation can be resolved and prevented by drinking enough water. Many laxatives work by drawing water into the bowels.

"Acid stomach" and heartburn can be due to not enough water.

Being properly hydrated helps with certain pains including muscle and colitis pains. Even anxiety attacks, hot flashes, and chronic fatigue can be attributed to not drinking enough water. Water can help lubricate joints which can decrease joint pain.

If you exercise, you need more water even if you didn't really sweat. Water evaporates from the skin and is exhaled during breathing.

Body fat and hydration level are inversely related. This means that if your body fat percentage is high, your hydration level is usually low. As you increase your hydration level, body fat usually reduces. This is why some people talk about "flushing fat out with water". The key isn't to drink gobs more water than we need, but to encourage proper hydration levels.

Poor hydration leads to water retention. If the body thinks it's not going to get enough water for the day because of poor water drinking habits, it will begin to store the water it is given. Fluids accumulate around areas with inflammation to buffer the body against it. When we drink enough water, we can keep flushing the extra fluids and some inflammation out of the body.

There are even conditions that can get worse when we don't drink water. These include aging (it speeds up), constipation, kidney stones, obesity, arteriosclerosis, glaucoma, diabetes, cataracts, hypoglycemia, and more.

What kind of water should we drink?

Water should be free from contaminants such as chlorine, fluorides, arsenic, heavy metals, pesticides, parasites, and any other dangerous substances.

The best water is well water that has been shown to be free from heavy metals, parasites, and pollutants.

If you don't have access to clean drinking water, invest in a reverse osmosis water filter for your home. If your home's water contains fluorides, bromine, or chlorine, install a charcoal filter in your shower head to prevent your skin or lungs from ingesting these while you clean yourself.

Check BookBonuses.NHWarriors.com for water filter suggestions.

Exercise

Our body was made to move. Moving our physical body has a beneficial effect on our internal organs and body systems.

What happens to a pond that is uncared for and just lies stagnant? Very quickly, algae, mosquitoes, and other undesirables take over. The same happens to our bodies internally when we don't exercise.

Walking and rebounding on a small trampoline are two great ways to move our lymph system. The lymph system is a waste transport system. It collects wastes and transports them for removal. This is why we often get a bad odor in our armpits if we don't use deodorant. There are key lymph nodes under our arms that dump wastes and bacteria. Strong body odor can indicate high body toxicity.

Because the underarm is a major lymph dumping site, we need to be sure that we don't use antiperspirants. This blocks the ability of the lymph to dump wastes which can lead to the lymph swelling. Painful, swollen lumps under the arm are a sign of blocked lymph. Discontinuing using antiperspirants has been enough for some people to be able to dissolve these lumps. There are ways to help the body break down and dissolve lumps like these for removal through the elimination channels.

Real Food

Our body thrives on nutrients. If we are overweight, we are probably eating too many macronutrients (fats, proteins, carbohydrates) and too few micronutrients (vitamins, minerals, phytochemicals, antioxidants, etc.).

Our body needs real food for fuel and information. Anything we ingest becomes information that directs how the body functions. What kind of information are you giving your body on a daily basis?

Real food doesn't include most items that come in a box, a foil bag, or a can. It also doesn't include most anything from a food joint with a drive-through.

Consider that most processed foods are also refined. This is a fancy word for stripping real food of most of its nutrients. When we strip food of vital nutrients, it provides negative nutrients. How is that possible?

Your body requires all the nutrients that a whole plant contains in order to process and digest it. When we strip that away, our body has to provide those missing nutrients, which we probably only have in short supply already.

To make us feel better about the stripping away of these vital nutrients, we see the word enriched on the label. In essence, enriched means that one or two of the stripped away nutrients have been added back. This is almost always done with inferior versions of what was taken away.

Refining a product is like a mugger in an alley taking away everything someone has on. Everything. They see them standing there cold, naked, and barefoot and take a little pity on them. So they enrich them by giving back their socks. Would that make you feel enriched?

Me neither.

Rest/Relaxation

A customer at my store asked me what I recommend for someone who wants more energy during the day or if they were feeling drowsy while driving. I recommended getting regular periods of rest during their week, slowing their life down, and getting enough nutrition and sleep.

We can't have consistent energy if we are always going and never resting. At some point, our bodies will break down.

If you are eating healthy foods, getting enough water, getting sufficient sleep at night, and making time for relaxation during your week and still suffering from low energy, I suggest you put some of the information in this book to use.

I really recommend against the use of stimulants. There is a reason your body is tired and worn out. It is probably due to a lack of nutrition and good supplements combined with a too-busy lifestyle. Using stimulants when we are stressed and burnt out is the very meaning of the phrase, "beating a dead horse". If you are stressed and tired all the time, it is better to support your body emotional and nutritionally and learn how to slow your lifestyle down. For many, this second option seems impossible. The 30 Day Change Anything Challenge included in this book will be especially helpful for this.

My favorite supplements for low energy are adaptogens. They contain nutrients that feed the adrenals and help the body to adapt and handle stress in a healthy way.

Stress will always make you tired and worn out, especially if you aren't providing extra nutrients during every season that you experience extra or a lot of stress. When you catch yourself feeling tired or stressed, try increasing the dose of a quality blend of adaptogenic herbs. One of my favorite blends includes alfalfa, ashwagandha, astragalus, eleuthero, kelp, Korean ginseng, reishi, schizandra, and suma. BookBonuses.NHWarriors.com

Emotional Peace

Can someone truly be healthy if they are in constant turmoil inside? I don't believe that is possible.

Our emotions and feelings create our thoughts. If you are feeling depressed, you will look around you for things, thoughts, and reasons to reinforce the depression. Our thoughts then stimulate the brain to create certain hormones. Can depression ever create a positive hormone? No. We feel worse physically to enforce the thoughts we are thinking which enforces the emotions we are feeling. It really is a vicious cycle.

When we feel the same way most of the time, it locks that feeling into our body. The same thing that can happen over time happens almost instantly when we undergo trauma. The emotion becomes trapped in our body.

We need to learn processes that can help us live in positive emotions more often, and they become our new emotional set point.

Many people stay stuck at a low emotional setpoint their entire lives because they don't have the knowledge or tools to change it. We'll explore the benefits of improving your emotions and ways to do so next.

Key Learning

We need fresh air and sunshine on a regular, frequent basis.

Headaches can be caused by not drinking enough water.

Our bodies are made of electrically charged particles.

When you think you are hungry and nothing sounds good, try drinking a glass of water. You might actually be thirsty.

Water is involved in nearly every body function.

Not drinking enough water can contribute to a lot of health issues.

We need to drink water free of contaminants and chemicals.

Exercise is important for health.

Food is information that our body uses to determine how to function.

If we are often tired, we may not be relaxing enough or consuming enough nutrients.

Our emotions can keep our health stuck where it is at.

Write down any other key points you want to remember.

8

Getting Started: The A B C Method

Do you want to be healed?

This is an important question to ask ourselves before we begin a health journey. Some people are not ready to give up their illness. It has become part of their identity.

You can easily tell who these people are by the way they talk about their health. They say things such as:

"I can't eat that, I have _____ (insert any intestinal/digestive issue)."

"I'm not able to workout, I have ____ (insert any pain disease)."

"I'm not able to do the things I used to love to do because I have ____ (insert disease)."

Notice the common words in those sentences? They all say, "I have." Their disease has become something they now own and carry with them like a badge of honor. How many times have you used a similar phrase?

Are you ready to let go of ownership of this disease(s)? Are you ready to separate it from yourself? Because that will require you to be a different person than you are now. You have to be willing to do different things and think different thoughts. You may need to completely change the way you live.

You need to claim your healing now before you can even see it. This requires choice and action.

In the Bible verses John 5:1-18 is a story of a man who was given a choice and required to take action in order to receive his healing. He had been lame for 38 years. He hung out with the other "diseased" and lame people at the pool of Bethesda.

Every now and again, the pool of Bethesda would "bubble up" because of an underground spring. The belief of the day was that an angel stirred up the water. if you were the first to touch the water after the angel "troubled it", then you would be healed.

This lame man had no one to help him get to the water. Because of his infirmities, others would always get to the water first.

Now Jesus comes along one day and asks this man, "Do you want to be healed?"

The man says, "Yes, of course. That's why I'm here. But I can't get to the water."

Jesus tells the man, "Take up your bed and walk."

If you had been lame for 38 years and someone says to you, "Grab your bed and move on out," you would call them crazy. How many excuses would come to mind as your first thought?

Remember all those things you tell yourself you would do if your disease were no longer attached to you? And if someone were to say to you, "Just go do what you love to do," you would have a myriad of excuses at the top of your mind for why you can't do them.

Those excuses stop you from being the person who can do those things you are desiring to do. I say all this out of love because I want to challenge you to be greater than your disease. You have to be greater than your disease in order to overcome it. Living with a disease goes hand in hand in living with the emotions of fear, grief, anxiety, regret, apathy, hopelessness, despair, guilt, blame, shame, misery, and humiliation. These are negative emotions that hold us down.

There is not a lot of room for those emotions when we are living in health. Living in health is living with courage, trust, hopefulness, optimism, acceptance, forgiveness, reason, understanding, love, joy, completeness,

GETTING STARTED: THE A B C METHOD

bliss, and peace. These are positive emotions that lift us up.

Every time that we use the words "I have" or "I can't" when we are talking about our disease, we are living in negative emotions. Do those words make you feel heavier when you use them? They pull you down and keep you where disease can live and flourish.

Jesus told the man to get up and walk. It was up to the man to step up in faith and claim his healing. He was told to take his bed with him; otherwise, it would be too easy to come back to reclaim his place by the pool and his illness.

We have to be willing to remove the crutches and things that will make it easy to fall back into our old habits of disease. If you are living in a state of disease, you cannot be who you are now and be healthy. If you woke up tomorrow in perfect health, you wouldn't have the thoughts, patterns, habits, or environment to maintain it. You would gradually slip back into the old you and reclaim your old illnesses.

This pattern of slipping back into old habits is very apparent in people who win the lottery. Overnight wealth doesn't change their poor money habits. In the same way, overnight health won't change your poor self-care habits. Your habits and your lifestyle determine your health.

My husband and I are volunteer coaches for an organization called Marriage Team. (As a side note, if you are married or thinking about getting married, get some coaching through MarriageTeam.org. Your marriage will only improve if you do the work as you go through their coaching. It's amazing.)

Back to my point, when my husband and I coached our first couple through Marriage Team, the wife had a lot of pain issues, depression, Fibromyalgia, and all those things that commonly go together. The scripture verse about the lame man in John 5 is mentioned in the Marriage Team material as well as the question Jesus asked, "Do you want to be healed?" The Marriage Team workbook then asks, ' Why would someone not want to be healed?"

Take a moment and ask yourself that. "Why don't I want to be healed?" If you are being honest with yourself, you will probably come up with several answers. The wife of the first couple my husband and I coached did. She said, "Then people will expect more from me. They won't be so quick to give me sympathy. I'll be expected to contribute more and do more."

What reasons can you come up with for not wanting to be healed? Take a moment and write them down. Now really look at them. Are you willing to give that up? Because if not, then nothing I or anyone else can teach you can help you. You have to be willing to be different. You have to be willing to get rid of the old you who carries this disease. "Take up your bed and walk."

That lame man would need to go get a job now because it wouldn't be so easy to be a beggar if people can see that he is a capable person. He had to get a different home. His old identity was gone. The people that he used to hang out with at the pool would no longer be in his life. He now had to be responsible for himself. Are you ready for this? If the answer is "no" right now, it's okay. I would suggest going through the 30 Day Change Anything Challenge in this book with a question similar to, "What would it take for me to be willing to be 'healthy'"?

Sometimes there are people we hang out with who are contributing to our illness. Or places we go. Or things in our home. Or our home itself. What are you willing to let go of in order to find the you that can be filled with vibrant health and energy?

Key Learning

Health will never be forced upon us; we have to truly want it.

We can't identify with our diseases if we want to be healthy.

Being healthy requires that we be a different person.

Negative emotions can hold diseases in our body.

Your habits and lifestyle determine whether you experience health or disease.

Do you want to be healed?

9

Activate: Opening the pathways

Have you ever gone through a storage unit that you've been piling things into for the last years or decades? Maybe it's not as big as a storage unit. It could be a room, a closet, or even a junk drawer. When you go through those things you are storing, how easy is it to get rid of things? "This item has sentimental value, I'll keep that." "I may use this someday; I should keep it." "I don't know what to do with this so I should just keep it."

Physical items are responsibilities that can weigh us down emotionally. We have to work in order to take care of them. My husband and I bought our house three years after we got married. I decided then that I didn't want anything that we couldn't store on our property (1.5 acres).

When we got married, we needed a storage unit because we were living in a small apartment. Within a year, that storage unit was upgraded to a larger size. When we purged the storage unit and got rid of a lot of stuff that was not contributing to the life we wanted, it was as if a great weight was lifted from my shoulders.

Things continually come into our lives. We have to work to only keep that which contributes to us. I was one of the first people in my circle to read the book about the Japanese art of decluttering. You touch every item you own and see if it makes you happy. If it doesn't, out it goes.

Anything that doesn't make you happy is contributing to your unhappiness.

There isn't really much in this world that is truly neutral. It's either positive or negative.

When we live in negativity, it is very difficult to get rid of things. Have you ever gone through your storage drawer, closet, room, or unit and been emotionally unable to get rid of anything? Instead, you just make a big mess, sneeze from all the dust, and pack it up essentially how it was and shut the door again. Now you feel defeated and worse than if you had just left it alone.

This is part of the process that can happen when we try to open up and get rid of things from the body. It can be uncomfortable, like a sneezing fit. It can get downright messy. And the more we have stuffed down and stored away in the body, the more difficult it is to get rid of it. The pathways to help the body move things out can get clogged in the same way that garbage bags get filled and shoved someplace when you don't know where to put it.

Opening up these pathways are some of the first things we need to do. The garbage has to be able to go someplace. If you are trying to clean out a giant storage unit and only have a tiny trash can to throw things away, it can be a long painful process that doesn't seem to get any forward momentum. We just keep stirring up dust.

Old Stories

What old stories do you tell yourself? "I'm fat. I'm unhealthy. I'm in a lot of pain. I'm tired all the time." Do you any of your stories sound like that?

If you are wanting to change any of those things, it needs to become yesterday's news. You can't keep talking about it in the present tense anymore.

Consider your favorite book, one that inspires you. What makes it inspirational? It's the journey and the change that the hero of the journey undergoes. They didn't become the hero of the story overnight. It's typically a long and arduous process from normal to hero. The more difficult their journey, the more we look up to them.

Are you ready to become the hero of your story?

All it takes is a decision to begin. Then start acknowledging and affirming to yourself that you are on your journey.

"I am becoming healthier every day. I am getting closer to my goals every day." This is how you remind yourself that you have begun your journey and refuse to be the old you who lived with pain and disease.

Opening the pathways

Have you ever collected things in your life without getting rid of an equal number of possessions? What you have just piles up until you have to get rid of things or get a storage unit?

This can happen in our body as well. I've already said that it takes nutrients, which most of us are sorely lacking in, in order for our body to be able to detox and take out the trash.

When we take out the trash, we usually gather it in a central location where we keep the garbage pail and ideally have a bag to hold it all in. Then we pull out the bag and walk it out to the trash bin. Once a week we put the trash bin at the curb and the trash is taken away. The process is easy if you have all the proper components.

But when our bodies get bogged down by trash and it can't get rid of, it all just accumulates as if we have no trash pail in our house, no bag to put it in, no door or window to throw it out and no trash collector or way to take it to the dump. It just collects and collects.

Our detox pathways can become so bogged down until they aren't even open for things to move out. Imagine living in a house where nothing ever gets thrown away (waste, even excrement, can't move out) but new things and trash come in and are created all the time.

We already talked about the four organs of elimination that need to be working. Those are the heavy lifters that function like the trash pail that collects and the trash bag that helps you take those things out.

But how do we get what needs to be eliminated to those organs? We need to open the pathways.

The most common bump in the digestive pathway sits right under the front of our ribcage. If we carry a lot of tension there, we can cause a hiatal hernia.

This is where the esophagus gets caught up in the diaphragm.

People with digestion issues, difficulty swallowing, and acid reflux often have difficulty in this area. We need to push the stomach down and away to correct this. This is something we can do manually over time. Taking some lobelia internally when working on this can help relax the muscles so they can cooperate.

A hiatal hernia and an inflamed ileocecal valve often go hand in hand. Rarely is one found without the other. An inflamed ileocecal valve is a big hiccup in the intestinal system.

Imagine your toilet backing up onto your kitchen counters where you prepare your food. That is the situation that is happening in your intestines when the valve is inflamed and stuck open.

The ileocecal valve is supposed to be a one-way connection from the small intestine into the large intestine. Inflammation essentially props that valve open. Bacteria and waste from the large intestine are then able to flow the wrong way back into the small intestine.

This can cause a lot of health issues and discomfort. It commonly leads to an overgrowth of the wrong bacteria in the small intestine.

We can manually work out this inflammation and help close this valve. Your ileocecal valve is located approximately halfway between your belly button and your right hip bone. It is only found on the right side of the body. Press around in this area and see if anything feels painful.

Some of my clients have had so much inflammation here that only the slightest pressure creates a lot of pain. Others only have mild pain. If there is any discomfort in this area, I would recommend daily self-massage of about five minutes once or twice a day until well after the pain or discomfort ceases.

I've had many clients who came to work with me frustrated because adhering to a strict diet plan and taking lots of supplements hadn't resulted in any improvement in their health. It is difficult to make progress when this valve is open.

I would recommend checking in with this valve on a monthly basis to assess for inflammation and help it move out. There is a video with more information about this in the member's area: BookBonuses.NHWarriors.com

Lymph

We need to support and work with our lymphatic system.

I know it doesn't always seem to work with us, such as in cases when our tonsils become inflamed time and time again. I understand that tonsillitis and strep throat is not fun, but it is really just the body sending out a warning sign asking for help.

I would use combinations containing many of the following herbs to support the lymphatic system: bayberry root bark, cleavers, capsicum, echinacea, garlic bulb, goldenseal, lobelia, mullein, plantain, prickly ash bark, red root, red clover, stillingia, yarrow.

BookBonuses.NHWarriors.com

There was an extensive study in Denmark done showing that people who had their tonsils removed were three times more likely to suffer from upper respiratory system diseases. Removing this important part of our immune system may do more long-term harm than ever realized.

I want to teach my clients to listen to their body and work with it not against it. Your body is doing the best it can. It is trying to keep you alive. Let's support it and assist it in its efforts.

Why a cleanse can make you feel sick.

So many people think they want to do a cleanse. It's a hip word in natural health. Yes, we need to cleanse But if your elimination pathways aren't open, then all a cleanse does is stir up the garbage and make you feel ill.

What good does it do to clean a house if you can't get rid of the garbage? It's like shaking your rug out in your living room. You are just stirring up the dust. Imagine how that would make you sneeze? Sneezing can definitely be a response to cleansing, especially if the pathways aren't open.

However, as we will talk about a little later, cleansing is very important and should be done on a regular basis.

Key Learning

Our detoxification pathways can become slow or even clogged.

Something either contributes to your happiness or unhappiness. Very few things are actually neutral.

Just like cleaning a house that has been shut up for years, opening up the bodies pathways isn't always a neat and tidy process.

We need to change the stories that we tell ourselves.

Are you ready to become the hero of your story?

We can manually address a hiatal hernia and an inflamed ileocecal valve.

Work with your body, not against it.

Write down any other key points you want to remember.

10

Activate: Elevated Emotions

Have you ever tried to pick up a helicopter? It is a heavy hunk of steel, but it has the ability to be weightless and fly. How is that possible? By spinning a propeller very quickly.

When I was growing up, my mother was a huge Lance Armstrong fan. She would watch hours of the Tour de France. Have you ever gotten on a bike and tried to make the wheels go that fast?

We climb on a bike and struggle to make the wheels go round and round, but it looks effortless for those people who race professionally.

The key is speed. Speed makes things lighter so much so that helicopters and other metal objects can fly.

Our emotions have a speed or a lack of speed to them. Guilt, shame, fear, apathy, even grief are all heavier emotions. They slow us down and weigh us down. Take a moment to think about something you feel ashamed of. Is that a light or heavy feeling?

Now think about someone you love and care about. Think of the joy of being around them. Is that lighter or heavier?

The emotions we live with most of the day determine our energy level for that day.

Have you ever had a day where you don't feel well, maybe you were in pain all day long. Nothing sounded good or interesting. You felt very apathetic and even sorry for yourself. There wasn't a lot you were able to bring yourself to do that day. We think that our physical body is causing the emotion, but emotions actually cause physical responses.

The next time you feel a negative, lower emotion, try to shake it off and notice where you feel discomfort in your body. That is where you are storing the emotion. That is why it comes back so easily. Your body has memorized it and has been storing it for a while.

You might try asking yourself if you are ready to let it go. Is it serving you? Does the emotion of apathy contribute to you and your life goals? If not, ask yourself if you are ready to let it go. When you have truly removed it from your body, that place will no longer hurt. This can take a lot of work, especially if you are new to emotional processes like this.

The body will hold on to the emotion if you are using it to protect yourself or if there is something you need to acknowledge about it. If you ask, "Am I ready to let this go?" and the answer is no, then you should ask, "What purpose is this serving?" Once you have learned the purpose, then usually you are able to release it.

When I was first introduced to the process of releasing negative emotions, I was skeptical as well. I wasn't sure how it was going to help me feel better physically.

Initially, I went through a process in a book called The Emotion Code. It's a wonderful book and there is a free app you can get on your phone for it. If you are interested in learning how to practice applied kinesiology, also called muscle response testing, on yourself or others, they have multiple explanations in the book. I won't go into that here as that book explains it very well.

After I had finished The Emotion Code process and reached a point where I had no more emotions that needed to be cleared from my body, there was an astonishing improvement to my PMS symptoms. Prior to that process, I struggled with my menstrual cycle.

It was never "normal". I had discontinued birth control after my husband got his vasectomy. This was an amazing relief for me as I didn't know then how to prevent an unwanted pregnancy with any other way except for taking chemicals and hormones that I didn't agree with taking.

I had already spent years improving my health and depression, but I still had difficult menstrual cycles. I knew these could be corrected naturally. I knew that PMS and menopausal symptoms are just a sign of toxicity in the body, but I hadn't figured out how to correct mine yet.

After I finished clearing the trapped emotions in my body, it was like a switch was flipped with my PMS issues. No longer did I have horrible cramping for a day or two at the beginning of my cycle. In fact, I no longer had cramping at all. The bleeding lightened and the length of my period shortened by a day.

This all happened practically overnight. One month was a rough period, the next was easy peasy.

Clearing emotions is something we need to do on a regular basis. And we need to utilize more than just one methodology. Not all of my health problems were solved miraculously by this, but I did eliminate one very bothersome symptom.

It has been over a year, and my menstrual cycles are still the easiest they have ever been in my life even when I was on birth control.

Tooth Infection and Clearing Emotions

Recently, I was going through a time of feeling really depressed. It was enough that my husband commented on it. I used another of my emotion clearing tools and asked if I was ready to release the depression.

When I went to do so, I noticed that the depression emotion I was feeling was sitting in my jaw. I had been struggling with a tooth infection for about six months. I adamantly refuse to take any more antibiotics in my life so I had been doing mega doses of vitamin c as well as making charcoal and essential oil pastes to put against the gums near the infected area.

Off and on for months, my gums in that area would be swollen. Then I would realize I was slacking on the amount of vitamin c I was taking and up the dose again. Some days I was taking 20-30 grams of vitamin c to try to get this infection under control.

Now please note that I am not advising you to deal with a tooth infection on your own in this way. They can definitely be very serious. I would advise you to go to the dentist. But I'm not about to take more antibiotics nor have any more conventional dentistry done because of the heavy metals they put in your teeth. Yes, I know they no longer use mercury amalgams. Now they are putting aluminum in your mouth and other dangerous metals. And all my teeth problems as an adult are related to fillings that I had as a child. I'm not about to let anyone drill on any more of my teeth. Okay, maybe the dentist rant is over now.

As I released the depression that had been sitting in my jaw, I was able to release the infection as well. It has been over a week that I have not been taking anything for the infection that was in my jaw and it continues to improve, the swelling is consistently decreasing, the pain is gone, and it feels fine.

I understand if you don't believe that story because it was mind-blowing to me and I'm the one who experienced it.

Does this mean that I won't ever struggle with depression again? Of course not. We are all humans. And we experience a wide variety of emotions and pick up emotions from each other all the time. But now I know what to do with that emotion when it does come back.

How do we actually release the emotion? It can be as easy as asking yourself if you are ready to let it go. There is often a noticeable feeling of lift afterward. You can feel that your body is not as heavy as it was just moments earlier.

Other tools I have used to help people clear and neutralize negative emotions are tapping or EFT aka emotional freedom technique, and NLP, neuro-linguistic programming. Utilizing a combination of the two, I have watched someone release anxiety to clear congestion instantly and also remove the anxiety in the way of making a job change decision.

Episode 14 of the NHWarriors vlog, which you can find on YouTube or Facebook.com/TirzahHawkinsHealth has about 30 minutes of tapping that you can follow along with. Once you know the points to tap on, you can follow along with your eyes closed.

One word of caution: I don't recommend watching a tapping video without tapping along yourself. It's too easy to retraumatize yourself. When you tap along with the video, you are neutralizing those emotions.

Key Learning

When something moves quickly, it becomes physically lighter.

Negative emotions weigh us down.

I utilized emotion clearing as talked about in the book The Emotion Code to eliminate my pms symptoms.

The emotional freedom technique (EFT or tapping) combined with Neuro-Linguistic Programming (NLP) is helpful for clearing trapped emotions from the body.

Write down any other key points you want to remember.

11

Activate: Emotional Clearing

To help you start clearing some emotions, I'm including a tapping script here. Customize it to yourself. Replace the descriptive words I use here with words that apply to you.

There are four acupressure places that you will tap on as you go through this script. The first is between the eyebrows. The second is the bony part at the side of your eye. The third is the bony part under your eye. The fourth is the soft flesh below the middle of your collarbone on either side of your body..

You can use as many fingers as you like to tap these places. Most commonly, people use two. Also, don't tap so hard that you injure yourself.

I've been working a lot with my friend Lynnette lately. She's going through some crazy life changes, getting out of an abusive 20-year marriage. I offered to do some tapping sessions with her to help with the anxiety she is experiencing.

I asked her, "What do you feel is the benefit that you are noticing from going in and working on these emotions?"

Lynnette: "I think one of the biggest benefits is to realize the emotions that are stuck for one and where in that lifetime, my lifetime, it's become stuck. There have been some recent events in my life that have brought in frustration, anxiety, anger, bitterness, resentment.

"Well, now I'm able to look back at an earlier age and realize that they had been there for that amount of time and the suppression of them.

"And then within my own children's lives as well. I have a younger son who's struggling with frustration, anger, and I see him now not dealing with them properly. And it's hard as a mom especially because you want to help them through that process of dealing with it and recognizing it and that they're okay to have. So that's probably the biggest."

Me: "A lot of us do that. We have this emotion or an event that happens in our childhood that is, it's bigger than us. We aren't able to deal with it. And in order to cope with it, we'll shove it down, and shove it into our bodies, and we'll carry it with us. We're then more likely to experience events that make us feel that way when we are carrying that emotion trapped inside of us. And now you're noticing, you're watching your children do that."

Lynnette: "Yes."

Me: "And realizing how detrimental it was what you did in your own childhood."

Lynnette: "Yes."

Me: "But it's really just a way for us to try to cope with something that's bigger than us."

Lynnette: "Yeah, exactly. Exactly. And I think that too you find it really difficult to find people to help you cope with it because we don't really know how. You stuff it away somewhere inside your body and it eventually comes back."

Me: "It comes back and then we use it as a crutch. We continue staying in that emotion. "Well, I had this traumatic event that happened to me, so I'm allowed to continue being a victim each time I want to play that card." We want empathy and sympathy because this emotion is still too big for us to deal with."

Tapping Script

Here is a tapping script for you to follow. Be sure to personalize it to yourself as much as possible. Use the locations in your body where you are feeling the emotion. Use your own words to describe how it feels.

You may want to record yourself reading the script so you can use it with your eyes closed. That often helps things shift faster as we disconnect from outside distractions and can focus on our bodies.

This script is centered around anxiety, but once you get a feel for it, you can go back and use it for any emotion.

Think of the earliest emotion that you can where you felt anxiety. I also have people think of the youngest age that they can imagine themselves having anxiety. This is especially beneficial if you can't remember a lot of your earlier memories.

Go ahead and bring to your mind a picture of yourself as young as you can feeling anxiety. If you can't remember a specific instance, that is okay. The younger you can imagine feeling that, the more helpful the process can be.

Step into that feeling at that early age. On a scale of one to 10, how strong can you make the anxiety feel? We want to start out with it really strong. Bring in as many details as you can that would make you feel anxious at that age until you can make the anxiety a 10.

Now notice where you feel it in your body. Notice the sensations there. I will include here some words and sensations my clients have used to describe their anxiety. Be sure to personalize it for yourself.

Begin by tapping between your eyes and say, "I release and let go all guilt."
Tap the side of your eye and say, "I release and let go all shame."
Under eye: "I release and let go all traumas."
Collarbone: "I release and let go all embarrassments."
Between the eyes: "I release and let go all fear."
Side of eye: "I release and let go all anxiety."
Under eye: "I release and let go all hurts."
Collarbone: "I release and let go all baggage."
Now grab your wrist. Take a deep breath in. Let it out. Say, "Peace."

Take a moment and go to some memory that makes your body feel really good. We all have at least one. It might be a location like a beach or a forest that makes you feel really good. It might be a memory of a time with a certain person that makes you feel really good. You might remember some accomplishment that makes your body feel good. You want to think of something that brings a smile to your face, that gives you a good shiver down your back, some really pleasurable thought or memory.

Find one and really notice how your body feels as you think about it. Bring it into color. Try to step into your body in the memory instead of just seeing yourself in your mind. Don't move on until you find this really good feeling because you are going to continue to use it throughout the rest of this tapping script. We'll keep returning to it.

Now go back to the earlier age and the feeling of anxiety. Feel it again in your body. Notice if it has shifted or lessened at all. Assess it again on a scale of one to 10. Most people find that it has changed a little and even reduced. In order to achieve a true change though, we need to keep working on it until it reaches zero.

Step back into that original memory; feel it again. Make it as big as you can, and let's resume tapping.

Between the eyes: "I release and let go this knot (replace with what you are feeling) in my gut (replace with the location you feel it).

Side of eye: "I release and let go the nausea."

Under eye: "I release and let go the helplessness."

Collarbone: "It's safe to let it go."

Between the eyes: "I release and let go this tightness."

Side of eye: "I release and let go the trauma."

Under eye: "I release and let go the tension."

Collarbone: "It's safe to let it go. I'm safe now."

Grab your wrist. Take a deep breath in; let it out. Say, "Peace." Return to that really good feeling thought or memory from earlier. Really feel it again. Bring the good feeling into as much of your body as you can. Bring the feeling into the top of your head, feel it run down your spine, down your legs, into your feet. Wiggle it into your toes.

When you are ready, return to that earlier age and the anxiety. Assess it again. How strong is it on a scale of one to 10? Has it shifted or moved? Does it feel different? Get a sense of what it feels like before continuing tapping.

Between the eyes: "I release and let go this knot in my gut."

Side of eye: "I release and let go this tension in my back."

Under the eye: "I release and let go this anxiety in my body.

Collarbone: "It's safe for my body to release it. My body can unwind now."
Between the eyes: "It's safe to relax."
Side of the eye: "Let it go."
Under the eye: "It's safe to let it go."
Collarbone: "I don't have to carry this anymore."

Grab your wrist. Take a deep breath in. Let it out. Say, "Peace." Return to that good feeling memory. Imagine yourself in that memory wrapped in your favorite comfort item. Feel that item against your skin. Now surround the entire memory with your favorite color. Run the good feeling like a gentle squeegee from the top of your head down to your feet.

When you are ready, go back to the anxiety memory. Take a moment to think about where it is sitting in your body, how strong on the scale it is, and what it feels like.

What in the memory is causing the anxiety? Typically at a young age, it is a person. We are afraid of what the person can do to us because we aren't old enough to protect ourselves. Who or what in the memory is causing the anxiety?

If you are a child in the memory, you may see the other person as much bigger than you. Whatever it is in the mental image you have that is causing the anxiety, I want you to skew the image so that you are way bigger than it is.

Shrink down what is causing the anxiety to really small. If it is an image, push it so far away from you that it is no bigger than a pinhead. If it is a voice, make it so quiet you can barely hear it. If it is a person, make them the size of a flea compared to you. You will find that you have control of what you see and hear in your mind. You can change and alter it. Get it really small or quiet, then begin tapping again.

Between the eyes: "I release and let go this image (or voice, person, etc)."
Side of the eye: "It is no longer bigger than me."
Under the eye: "It no longer has control of me."
Collarbone: "It no longer haunts me."
Between the eyes: "I am so much stronger than I give myself credit for."
Side of the eye: "I no longer need to react to this."
Under the eye: "It is safe to let this go."

Collarbone: "I release and let it go."

Grab your wrist. Take a deep breath in; let it out. Say, "Peace." Go back to that really good memory and sit with it for a bit. Feel the comforting item you brought in. Wrap yourself with your favorite color. Feel the color like a loving presence around you.

Bring in your favorite song or music. Really hear the beat or the lyrics. Stay with that for as long as you want.

When you are ready, return to the anxiety and early memory. Notice how it has shifted and decreased. Those of you whose bodies are ready to let things go may not be able to find any anxiety at this point.

In the beginning, it would take me about thirty minutes of tapping before my body would have a release. After a while, it only took fifteen minutes. Then five. Now it can sometimes happen for me in just the few seconds it takes to acknowledge the emotion and ask it to leave.

I'm going to assume that some of you reading this are new to tapping and aren't able to release trauma and emotions as easily as those who are practiced at it. For that purpose, I'm going to include two more rounds here. If that still doesn't release the anxiety, you can continue from the top and loop through the script as much as you need to. Keep replacing the specific feelings and locations to apply to you.

Now if you were holding a cup of water and poured it into the ocean, how much of your original water could you get back? (Questions like these help break up our typical thought patterns.)

Go back and feel into any anxiety left and begin tapping between your eyes: "I release and let this go."

Side of eye: "It happened so long ago."
Under eye: "I don't need to keep traumatizing myself with it."
Collarbone: "I don't have to hold myself hostage any longer."
Between the eyes: "I don't have to be hurt by this anymore."
Side of eye: "I'm only hurting myself. This memory only affects me now."
Under eye: "I can free myself. It's safe to free myself."
Collarbone: "It's safe to be myself. It's safe to be free."
Between the eyes: "It's safe to let this go."

Side of eye: "I am free now."
Under the eye: "I've learned what I needed to from this."
Collarbone: "And now it is safe to let the trauma and anxiety go."
Grab your wrist. Deep breath in. Let it out. Say, "Peace."

One more time feel into the memory and the anxiety. Feel where it is in your body. Rate how strong it feels.

Between the eyes: "I release and let go all trauma associated with this memory."
Side of eye: "I don't need it anymore."
Under the eye: "The memory of it is fading. I'm going to choose peace instead."
Collarbone: "It is safe to be me. It is safe to be happy. It is safe to feel peaceful in my life."
Grab your wrist. Take a deep breath in. Let it out. Say, "Peace."

Once the strong negative emotion has been neutralized, and you go back to the memory, most people picture themselves just sitting or standing doing nothing. Because you control the movies you play in your mind, I want you to take yourself at whatever age you were as we were releasing the emotion and visualize yourself doing something you really love to do. Swimming, playing, making mud pies, playing dress-up. Visualize yourself doing that and really enjoy it for a moment.

It's quite common for the original emotion and the feelings in the body it triggers to move from one location to another during the course of the tapping. It can settle into multiple places in the body. If you are someone who struggles with the same emotion like anxiety a lot, it can be helpful to go through this process many, many times working through different memories and ages. The earlier the age you work on, the more impactful it is.

Don't stop a tapping session until you have neutralized the emotion to a zero, where you can't find it anymore. Then go through the process of picturing yourself doing something you loved to do at that age.

It is quite common to feel relieved and lighter at the end of this process. You'll begin to feel different the more you practice doing this. It is also common to cry as you release old emotional traumas. Be gentle with yourself during this process.

After her first session with me, Annalyse had this to say, "After just one emotional clearing session, I'm not entirely convinced that my diagnosis of Fibromyalgia, autoimmune, and heart diseases, are actually true. Or even actually there.

"I think the majority of my pain, if not all of it, is emotional pain that's festered itself so deeply into all of my systems. Whether it be unforgiveness or trauma or any other unresolved emotions that are disguising themselves as Fibromyalgia, POTS, or any of the other things I have. I'm very excited to continue this journey and see where it takes me."

Emotional work is one of the best places to start when working on our health. We can accomplish positive changes by just doing this work alone.

If you are interested in more emotional clearing work, you can subscribe to my emotion clearing library at Emotions.NHWarriors.com

Flower Essences

Negative emotions are a warning sign that something is wrong; they are harmful to our soul the way that physical pain is a sign of damage being done to our physical body. These may include feelings such as anger, sadness, guilt, depression, anxiety, and shame.

Convention medicine doesn't teach us how to deal with the cause of them. Conventional medicine is also called allopathic medicine which means "against the symptom"; it only fights the symptoms.

I need to teach you how to address the cause. If a damn breaks and water floods your town, is it better to try to continually remove the water or work to rebuild the damn stronger and better than it was before? If you only address the over present incoming water, then you don't ever get anywhere.

One of the most difficult things I have to get those who come to me for help with their health to understand is that natural healing is not about symptomatic relief. That isn't truly healing. It is about addressing the source. Just like physical issues, we need to address the source of emotional stress as well.

We can discover what is causing our emotional distress and address it rather than masking the pain with prescription or recreational drugs, alcohol, sex, addictions, staying busy all the time, being a workaholic, etc.

We can take responsibility for our own emotional well being instead of taking out our emotions on others through jealousy, attacking, or playing the victim.

Our emotions are caused by how we choose to respond to certain situations. We need to understand that we have a choice. When we choose the same reactions over and over again, they become habitual and build our personality.

I need you to understand that if you want to heal your body, the work that needs to be done is on both a physical and an emotional level. You will need to start practicing healthier physical and emotional patterns until you become a healthy personality, which equates to a healthy person.

Many stories have been told of prisoners of war and concentration camp prisoners whose spirits were never broken. These people understood that only they had control over their thoughts, emotions, and reactions. No one could take that freedom from them.

Flower essences are a tool that works on a vibrational level similarly to the way that homeopathics work. They can help to break up toxic energy patterns in the body so that negative emotions can be brought to the surface and released. They are useful in conjunction with energy clearing, nutritional supplementation, and herbal detoxification and are not a substitute for any of them.

Properly prepared flower essences from a reputable company can be completely non-toxic and able to be given to people of all ages including infants as well as pets.

I recommend to all my clients that they take a flower essence blend appropriate to their personality for at least the first three months of them beginning to follow the Natural Health Warriors Protocol.

If you would like to find the flower essence blend appropriate for you, you can find a link to a quiz in the book bonuses members area: Book-Bonuses.NHWarriors.com

Key Learning

Negative emotions can physically slow us down and make us experience low energy.

Negative emotions can become trapped in our body and contribute to disease.

I (Tirzah Hawkins) personally resolved my menstrual issues by clearing negative emotions from my body.

We often suppress emotions we don't know how to deal with as children. This can lead to emotional and physical issues later in life.

Tapping or EFT (Emotional Freedom Technique) is a useful tool for helping to clear negative emotions that have become stuck in a person's body.

Flower essences are helpful for helping to break up and release negative emotional patterns in the body.

12

30 Day Change Anything Challenge

I want to introduce you to a process that you can use to change things you are unhappy with in your life. It's designed to help you see that you have more control over your life than you would imagine, and you have a multitude of choices about most things in your life.\

I find a lot of depression connected to people who think they have no choices. They believe that they are stuck. They never wonder how life can get any better because they believe that it can't.

Think of some things in your life that you are unhappy or dissatisfied with: anything that you want to be better. Throughout this book, you'll find suggestions for things you can use this process to change.

Are you open to the places in your life that feel stuck changing in a way that you haven't even thought of yet? If I were to ask you how those things could change, you might say "it can't" or just give me one or two options.

We grow up being given one or two choices. Do you want chocolate or vanilla? Some of us go crazy and rebel by picking the chocolate/vanilla swirl when given that option.

Remember that wonderful ice cream shop that had thirty-one flavors of ice cream? There are now way more than thirty-one flavors of ice cream ever created. Can you accept that there are more than thirty-one different options for each of the things in your life that you are dissatisfied with? There are more than we can count.

We often can't see that because we are emotionally stuck in the situation. Pick one of the items on the list that you want to change. Why haven't you changed it?

For instance, someone who wants to change their weight might tell me, "I don't exercise enough," or "I don't eat right" or "I have low thyroid.

Or if you have a difficult relationship with your spouse, you might say, "They don't listen to me" or "They are so stubborn" or "All they want is sex".

Notice how our first response to why something hasn't changed is to come up with excuses? Excuses are limitations. They are the walls to the little boxes we create to fit our lives in that limit what is possible.

Are you willing to do something incredibly simple in order to improve something in your life? It will take less than five minutes of your time each day. Plus, you get support throughout the whole process by joining the support group. When you work with a group to accomplish a goal, you are much more likely to succeed. Find a link to the group at BookBonuses.NHWarriors.com

Brainstorming

Before I introduce you to the process, I need to teach you the rules of brainstorming. Who knew there were rules for that, right?

Brainstorming is about getting the most possibilities, options, or choices on paper. We are looking for quantity, not quality. Even the silly choices get written down. Then, when we can't think of anything else, we ask: "What else?"

You don't get to evaluate the options when you are in the brainstorming process. All ideas are included right now. I encourage you to use a notepad on your phone or keep one in your purse at all times for writing down what comes to you throughout the course of these thirty days.

When you can't think of any more, you start asking yourself questions to bring out more ideas such as, "What would be the silliest option here?", "What would my brother, mother, uncle, child, etc. suggest I do?", "What would be the best option for all involved?" Keep asking and writing down the answers.

The Process

The process is as simple as finding ONE thing you want to change and stick with it for the 30 days. You may want to make a list of the other things that come to your mind when you think about doing this and record them for later.

Look at that one thing and notice how you feel about it. Does it make you unhappy, mad, frustrated, dissatisfied? Really get a sense of how you feel about it. Then acknowledge that. Say out loud, "I'm really unhappy (or insert your emotion here) about this. I'm open to other options."

Then repeat one of these questions or use them both in combination 30 times a day for 30 days: "How can this get any better?" or " What else can I choose?"

You can say these aloud when you are driving in your car, when you are taking a shower, when you go for a walk, or just sitting quietly before bed. It really doesn't take much time.

If spending five minutes to change something in your life for the better sounds like too much, are you really ready for a change? All change requires something of us.

How much energy are you willing to devote to the changes you say you are desiring? By choosing to purchase and read this book, you are acknowledging that you want a change in your life.

Reading a book requires a very small amount of energy which means that reading alone will effect a very small change. Application of what you have read is where you will begin to see results.

Because this process is so simple, many of the people reading this will dismiss the process. Don't be one of those people. They are making the choice, consciously or subconsciously, that this won't work because it is too easy. You can make a different choice. What could it hurt?

One of the biggest keys here is to look back over the rules of brainstorming. You don't get to discount or judge any answers that come to your mind for the 30 days. They all get recorded, even the ones that are immoral, illogical, or illegal. I'm definitely not encouraging you to do something immoral, illogical, or illegal. Please don't misunderstand that. This is just about getting more options than you ever thought possible down on paper.

My husband and I were introduced to the rules of brainstorming from an organization we volunteer for called Marriage Team. (If you are married or thinking about getting married, I highly recommend their marriage coaching. It can improve your relationship whether it is struggling or amazing already.)

One of the couples that my husband and I coached through the Marriage Team process has utilized some of the silly ideas that they came up with during their brainstorming processes such as having a truth or dare date night and even prank calling a relative. Don't discount any idea right now.

The easiest way to keep track of how many times you asked the question is to get a little tally app on your phone. You ask the question and hit a button. Ask the question; hit the button. It's as easy as that.

What do you want to change then? Do you have ONE thing? Write it down. You may initially read through this chapter in one sitting. If you do, be sure to return to it and work through it for the full 30 days in order to derive benefit from it.

For many people, especially those who have felt helpless, hopeless, without choices, or even as a victim in their life, this process may be the most important part of this book for you. You may go through the process several times before you begin to see the huge value it can contribute to you.

Day 1

I am _____ (dissatisfied, unhappy, etc.) with _____ (fill in the blank). What else can I choose? How can this get any better?" You don't have to repeat the statement 30 times, but I would recommend saying it each day at least once in conjunction with the questions so you remember and get the feeling of what you are working on.

You need to make the conscious decision that you are open to having another choice here, one that may be better than anything you can think of right now.

Don't say, "This won't work" or "Nothing will work". That kills all the possibilities before they have the chance to germinate. It may be helpful to acknowledge "I am open to something better. I am open to an option better than anything I thought was possible here."

Day 2

I initially announced this challenge as part of one of my podcasts and then posted it in my online group. I think it is important for anyone to be able to go through.

The benefit to me announcing it before I wrote this was that I noticed that people thought they were going to choose something to change, decide how to change it, and then commit to that plan for 30 days.

For instance, Rebekah wanted to work on getting more sleep and was going to try to go to bed earlier. Forcing yourself to do something you don't want to do for thirty days requires a lot of will-power, something we have a limited supply of each day.

I don't want my clients to have to rely on a lot of willpower. I want to teach them how to bypass that in order to make healthy changes easier. When we release the resistance that is causing us to behave in a certain way, we can naturally make a healthy change.

There are thousands of solutions to any given problem: we just haven't consciously acknowledged more than a handful.

It can help to go to the real thing, the core thing, you are dissatisfied with by asking, "Why is that important to me?" Rebekah thought she wanted more sleep at night. Why is that important? Because she wants to have more energy during the day. Why is that important? Because she has a lot of kids and home matters to take care of. Feeling like she has the energy to take care of her family might be closer to what she wants to work on through this process.

Examine what you wrote down and ask the importance of it. You may need to find a deeper issue, not the superficial thing. Ask "why is that important to me?" in response to each answer you get seven times in a row to find the real thing that is important to you to change. It can be helpful to have a friend or someone you trust ask you that question seven times.

Kendra wanted to record everything she ate for 30 days. Was she really dissatisfied with her lack of food recording? Or is she dissatisfied with her food choices? Or the way her body looks and feels? We need to go a little deeper. Maybe she is dissatisfied with the way she feels about her body. What is the real issue?

Now ask, "What else can I choose regarding this? What would be a better choice than the choices I am currently making?" 30 times a day for 30 days.

Why all this repetition? Because we need to ask our master processor and cataloger in our brain, the thing that records the millions of bits of data we are exposed to every moment, our subconscious, to bring us different answers.

When you are deciding what to eat for dinner, your subconscious will give you a few of your normal choices. That's why you only think about eating burgers or tacos. Haven't you been to a restaurant before? How many different things have you seen on all the different menus? How many recipe searches have you done online? How many pictures of amazing food have you pinned? Your subconscious records all of this.

But when we ask, "What should I have for dinner?" we are only given a few options. We typically can't handle more than that. Why? Because you don't want to have to decide between every single food dish you have ever seen, heard, or read about, appetizing or unappetizing each time you decide to eat.

Remember that Indiana Jones movie where they go to that awful temple that sacrifices people? Do you really want your brain to suggest eyeball soup or live snakes when you wonder what you should have for dinner? I definitely don't. Your subconscious filters for you. Sometimes it does it's filtering job way too well.

Your subconscious only presents you with the top options, one that you will probably choose because you choose it quite often. But that means that we just eat the same things over and over and over. We need to break out of these patterns, especially in areas where we make the same choices over and over again, that only lead us to unhappiness.

This is about exploring those other possibilities. Don't make a choice yet because you don't have very many options on the table. Just get to the real thing that you want to choose differently about for right now.

The first rounds of choices you get aren't really going to be helpful. You've probably explored them before. If you try to choose one of them again, you'll probably get frustrated. If there is one that you like, don't choose it now. Look at it and ask, "What would be even better than that option?" "What else is there to choose from?"

Try not to answer the question consciously. Let's make this supercomputer that is our mind work for us.

Day 3

Don't get stuck in judgment. Judgment is an idea killer. It creates limitations. Anything that we hold a judgment about is limited in its potential to be beneficial for us.

Have you ever asked a child for their ideas about a problem? Keep asking a five-year-old, "What else can you think of?" and they probably won't ever stop coming up with ideas.

As we get older, we start to judge things based upon other people's opinions of them. Ask a teenager to help you solve a problem, and they'll have far fewer ideas than the five-year-old.

Why? Because a teenager doesn't want to give you a silly solution or a dumb solution or a crazy solution. They care about the judgment you place on the response they give you. Most five-year-olds don't have that awareness of judgment yet.

Now if you were asking a five-year-old for their ideas and, after each one, you told them your judgment of it, would they reach a point at which they won't want to give you any more ideas? They'll eventually tell you, "I don't want to tell you any more; you just say all my ideas are dumb."

This is what happens when we judge the ideas that our subconscious gives us. We get the familiar ones first. "Okay, what other ideas do you have for me to choose from?" Then we get the less chosen. "Okay, what can be even better than that?"

At some point, we will start to get some completely new things. When you start to judge them, you shut down the creative, problem-solving process immediately. When you judge the ideas that come to you, you are judging yourself because you thought of the idea. You don't want to feel judged by yourself; therefore, you never allow yourself to think of new ideas.

Can you let go of that judgment right now? There are no silly ideas. There are no good ideas. There are no dumb ideas. There are no brilliant ideas. There are just ideas and options right now.

Labeling something as good or positive is giving it a judgment just as much as labeling it poor or bad. If we judge and say "Oh, that's a really good idea", we may be limiting ourselves to only coming up with ideas similar to that.

How should we respond then? To every idea that comes up, they are neither good nor bad; they are interesting. "Well, that's an interesting idea. What else is there?" "That's an interesting idea. What could be even better than that?" "What can be even more satisfying than that?" "What is the most awesome idea I can think of?"

When you think of a most awesome idea, don't label it as such. Just keep asking "What can be better than that?"

Day 4

How often do you thank yourself? Your body needs to know that you appreciate and feel gratitude for it. If you don't appreciate it, how do you expect anyone else to?

I believe that self-love is important. Remember the Bible verse that says, "Love your neighbor as you love yourself". To me, this means, you can only love your neighbor as much as you love yourself. If you have no love for yourself, can you truly love anyone else?

Hopefully you have a list of ideas at this point. Now it isn't necessary to sit and ponder the question waiting for answers. Ask the question. Repetition is helpful. Ask it 30 times each day. Then go about your day or go to sleep and let the answers come to you. Did you know you can send your brain to work for you, and it can perform for you while you sleep? Instead of skimping on sleep, thinking you are being lazy, give your brain a problem to solve and plenty of time to do it while you rest your body. When you are asleep is when your brain is most active.

Then when an idea comes to you acknowledge that your brain has been going to work for you. Start thanking your brain for working for you. When was the last time you thanked yourself for something? As silly as it may feel in the beginning, thank yourself for the new idea, record it, and say, "What else? What can be even greater than that?"

Day 5

Have you thought about how helpful it might be to stop judging things in other areas of your life? Or how you telling people your judgments about things they are considering in their lives that are limiting their possibilities?

When my husband was growing up, he told his sister that he was going to build a spaceship out in the garage that would fly him to the moon. His sister begged his mom, "Please tell him that isn't possible. Tell him he can't do that."

My husband loves to fly and wants to be a private pilot. At an early age he was told that because of his poor eyesight, he would never be allowed to get his pilot's license. Guess what? With the advancement in technology called LASIK eye surgery, he is now able to get a pilot's license.

Just because something is true for you doesn't mean it is true for someone else. Just because you think something is a bad idea doesn't mean it isn't right for someone else.

How many times have people passed judgment on something in your life so you decided not to even try? How many times have people passed judgment on something in your life, and you proved them wrong?

We've all seen someone get into a relationship we thought was wrong for them, and then we judged that it wouldn't last. I made that judgment about someone getting married, and they are still married almost 20 years later!

I had family members pass judgment when my husband and I bought our gym or the retail health store. I might not be writing this book if we had listened to the people around us telling us we were making mistakes by purchasing either of them.

Be open to possibilities and keep asking for greater ones.

Day 6

Can you catch (and stop) yourself when you begin to judge yourself? All this talk about judgment has me thinking of another Scripture verse, "Judge not, lest ye be judged."

Growing up, I had to memorize verses for school. The correspondence school I was enrolled in only used King James' Version. All the scriptures I know by heart are in old English like that.

No one likes to be judged. We immediately feel like we need to protect or defend something when we are judged. How often are we doing that to ourselves? Is it possible that part of the intention of this Bible verse is saying, "Don't judge yourself because it isn't good for you"?

Why do we feel the need to let someone else know that we think they are wrong? If you want more options in your life you have to quit judging the ones you have.

A lot of people say they want the best for their kids. Who determines what is best? Is what the parents wants the best? Or is what the child wants the best? Is what you want for your friend the best? Or is what your friend wants the best? Is there really one "best"?

We are meant to be creative and problem solvers. What if Thomas Edison had judged himself as a failure after the first attempt at the light bulb? What about the tenth? What about the hundredth? If he had stood in judgment of himself, would he have created something so incredible that we take for granted today? I'm thinking not. I'm sure he asked himself far more than 30 times for longer than 30 days, "What else is possible here? What am I missing to make this work? What would make this even better?"

Whether or not you give up or judge yourself affects those around you, maybe even as much as Thomas Edison's light bulb affects you today.

Day 7

We all have down days. I mean, aren't we all human? We can help ourselves through these slumps faster by allowing ourselves to recognize that we are experiencing an emotion.

Emotions aren't bad. They are just an indication of what our body is feeling.

It is helpful to know that an emotion doesn't need to define you. You are more than your emotions. They don't need to trap you either. We can learn to work with our emotions rather than against them.

When you find yourself dealing with an e-motion that you don't like or is on the list of negative emotions, allow yourself to feel it for a minute. Whether it is fear, guilt, anger, jealousy, acknowledge what you are feeling and allow it.

Don't sit in judgment of yourself that you are feeling that way. Instead, have an "That's interesting that I'm feeling _____" attitude. You can either choose to sit with the emotion, but I would suggest asking yourself, "What else can I choose? What would feel a little bit better than this?"

Some people get trapped in the idea that they can jump from shame, guilt, or anger to happiness in the flip of a switch. Those two emotions are so far apart. That is like working in an office in New York and stepping outside on your lunch break and being in Los Angeles. It's physically impossible. We can however work in New York and look at a picture of Los Angeles and allow it to help us feel a bit better. Then we can pretend we are in L.A. and feel another step better.

It's like being in poverty one moment and having millions of dollars the next. That isn't often how it happens.

We need to work our way up from lower emotions to the next higher one. The next time you are stuck in a negative emotion, take a moment to ask, "What would feel just a little bit better than this?" That is the feeling or emotion you want to reach for, not one that is worlds apart from where you are now.

Day 8

Are you still with us in this process? If so, you have completed seven days, and it's time for a little celebration. Don't stop though, and don't start evaluating your progress and ideas. You've been stuck in the same ruts and patterns for so long, it will take longer than a week to turn it all around. This is just the tip of the iceberg as far as ideas go. You may not even have many that you've never thought of before at this point. Don't worry; the good ones are coming. Just keep at it.

The best ideas might not even come to the surface until close to day thirty when you've got the clutter out of the way and your mind has accepted that it isn't going to be judged for giving you ideas you've never consciously thought of or considered yet.

Even if you think you have a winner, I encourage you to stay the course. Look at your favorite ideas and say, "I like this idea. But what can be even better? What can I choose that would be even better than this?"

Day 9

What has been the most difficult part of this so far? I'd love for you to share with us in the support group. (Find the link in your member area: BookBonuses.NHWarriors.com)

There are lots of things that are difficult for some people while being easy for others. Collaborating in a group allows multiple people to share ideas of what works for them.

Whenever it gets tough to stay consistent, I encourage you to look back on why this is important enough to you that you want something different.

Spend a little time daydreaming about a perfect solution: one that makes everyone involved much happier. Just be sure that when you are done, you keep asking the question, "How can it get even better than that?"

I can't wait to hear about all the answers coming to you. "That's interesting. What else would be even better?"

Day 10

Maybe it's time to let you in on a little secret. I hope this doesn't derail you from your path, but this holds true for the rest of the information in the book as well.

The circumstance in your life that you are working on in these 30 days might not be the biggest change that comes from this.

You may be what changes. Maybe you find a peace about the situation, or a new attitude, or a different way of looking at it. When you change, your situation changes.

An EFT practitioner I was learning from told about a client of his who was having relationship difficulties with her husband. Of course, she believed the problem was entirely his and the way he behaved.

She scheduled for them both to see the practitioner for EFT sessions. Hers was first, and his was the subsequent day. The day before his appointment happened, but after she had gone to hers, she wondered what they had done to her husband. He was a completely different person. In actuality, she was the one who had changed.

People respond to us differently when we change. And we can't force anyone else to change.

If you remain who you are now, then your life will stay as it is now. Your health and wealth and happiness will remain the same. People will treat you the same. If you want your life to be different, you need to decide that you are willing to be different than you are now.

What will you choose? The choice is completely up to you. But there are many more choices here than just yes or no because a choice to be different can look any way you want it to.

"What else can I choose? What would be even better than that?"

Day 11

Just a little continuing thought from yesterday: do you realize how much changing yourself changes how people respond to you?

Rather than punishing others for not behaving how we want them to, we have to focus on ourselves. What is the part of our behavior that is causing unwanted reactions from someone else?

Sometimes, when we quit holding something over someone else, they begin to behave differently towards us. When we quit reacting in a way that gives them their desired response, we take all the fun out of it for them.

How do people respond to someone in rags as opposed to someone in a lovely dress? Beyond their outward appearance, they are both being someone completely different. You have the power to decide how you want to be perceived.

"That's interesting. What else can I choose?"

Day 12

Even though we are more than one-third of the way done here, you may be tempted to get a little distracted at this point. Don't stray. Don't pick another topic. Focus on just one for the full 30 days. You haven't come close to thinking of all your choices yet. While you won't get there in just 30 days, because we can't ever find ALL our choices about anything, we can still find what is better than what we already have thought of consciously.

Let's stick this out together and expect something wonderful at the end. Something even better than what you've thought of so far. Changes take time, and this will be worth it.

Maybe it's time to say, "That's interesting. What is something even better that I can choose?

Day 13

Follow the good feeling. As I said at the beginning, a lie may be holding this in place, keeping you stuck. Lies feel heavy. Negative emotions feel heavy. They actually slow our body down and its energy field and processes down.

"The truth will set you free." Truth feels lighter. Positive emotions such as willingness, acceptance, love, joy, and peace all feel lighter. They increase the available energy in your body.

Have you ever noticed when you are sick, or dealing with a chronic illness, that if something comes along that brings love, laughter, and positive excitement, you find you have the energy to participate? This can be said even of people who are dying.

The lighter emotions create more energy in the body. Living with positive emotions more often can even help keep us from getting sick. Have you ever heard, "Laughter is the best medicine"? Well, that is mostly true.

Let's rise above our funk, reach for a good feeling, and say, "That's interesting. What else can I choose."

Day 14

Stop trying too hard. This isn't something you need to put effort towards. If you are experiencing any frustration around this, I encourage you to not expect an answer when you ask the question.

Right now, your subconscious mind might trust you as much as a feral kitten. We can't demand that a scared kitten come out and trust us Right Now. We need to be sweet and soft with it; then in time, it learns to trust.

You've probably been dissatisfied with that thing you are looking for more options for, for a very long time. You allowed it to be in your life until you reached a point that you decided you can't stand it for another minute. You can't remove a twenty-year-old oak tree, roots and all, in just a moment. What you have in this moment is the ability to decide that you will start the process to remove it and see it through. There aren't many truly amazing things in our lives that happen overnight.

No one gets married overnight, unless it was an arranged marriage or a vacation fling. How often are those amazing in the long-term? No one graduates from college overnight. We didn't get where we are overnight, and we won't get out of it overnight. But, if we are dedicated to change and improving ourselves, then we will wake up one morning in a much better place.

Take a little time to sit and appreciate knowing that you have choices. So many of them. For today, as you ask the question aloud, don't demand an answer. Just appreciate the question. How does the question feel to you? Like so many exciting possibilities? Like joy, peace, or fun?

Let's let it feel good. Even if just for today. "What else can I choose? What would be even better than anything I've thought of already?"

Day 15

Let's apply a little twist to the question for today and see which feels better.

Before we get to the new question, I want to keep encouraging you to check in with how something feels to you. Remember that if something is not true for you, it feels heavy. The truth feels lighter. This is just one of the ways you can begin to communicate with your body.

"What else is possible that I haven't thought of already?" You may have pages of answers so far, but there are still endless possibilities. How many are you willing to receive?

We always have choices, but we often blind ourselves from them. Even a little bit of stress can block creative thinking.

"What would I choose if I wasn't worried about what others would think of me? What would I choose if I could make any choice I wanted?"

One of my clients was struggling with living in an abusive situation for years. She was trying to decide if it would be worth it to stay in the situation for her kids. Since she couldn't really see a way out, she contemplated suicide.

When she and I would talk, I would tell her some of the most obvious choices that came to my mind. She couldn't always wrap her head around them because she was in stress and survival mode.

If you find yourself unable to see more options and more choices for the situations in your life that stress you out the most, try utilizing tapping, flower essences, or other emotional clearing work to neutralize the panic in order to begin allowing your brain to work again.

Continue the rest of the challenge with whichever question feels best or alternate them by day.

Day 16

What's with all these feelings, energies, heaviness, and lightness that you keep talking about? Good question.

When I first started studying natural health, I was stuck on the parts of the body that we would study in anatomy class. My thought was if I can get the organs and glands working correctly, then that will "fix" the problem the client came to see me for. That's just the tip of the iceberg.

We create a heaviness in our life around anything that isn't working for us that kind of locks it into place. Because it becomes so heavy nothing moves it.

I discovered that some of the afflictions we deal with start with an emotion or trauma. The disease or symptom then festers and becomes apparent over time, often with the person experiencing it having no known correlation between an event and the symptoms it causes.

We have to "lighten the load" in order for these things to budge. That is the point of this work. Are you willing to spend a simple five minutes a day to find greater possibilities for your life? Seems too easy doesn't it?

This isn't a New Year's resolution. This is doing something small and simple to find a better future for ourselves. And a better future for us, affects those who are closest to us.

What an interesting thought. "What else can I choose?" Carry on.

Day 17

I wanted to expound on how your life affects those closest to you. And it has nothing to do with physical proximity. By helping yourself, you are helping the people around you as well. Good and bad habits are contagious. As you discover and begin acting upon your new choices, you are helping others around you see that they have other choices they can make as well.

A 32-year study collaborated on by Harvard University and the University of San Diego showed how obesity was contagious between people in a close relationship. It didn't matter if the close friend or family member lived next door or on the other side of the globe either.

The study showed that if you had a close friend become obese, you were 171% more likely to become obese as well.

Do you want to be spreading good or bad habits to your close relationships? Start by choosing to change the things you want to change in your life. Put on your oxygen mask first.

If that feels difficult, ask, "What can I choose that will help me get what I want in the easiest way?"

Day 18

What are you trying to protect yourself from? We all have areas in our life that we create neat little boxes around. These boxes prevent us from looking out and seeing the other possibilities. There are ALWAYS other possibilities.

Take a moment to ask yourself: "What is the purpose of this box? What is it protecting me from? What rules is it helping me to abide by? Does this box limit me in a good way? Does the box limit me in a bad way? Am I ready to let myself out of the box? Did I realize it was there in the first place? Can the box go away now?"

Oftentimes we can help ourselves out of our boxes by realizing they are there and acknowledging the reason we put up the box in the first place. We only create limitations because we think they will protect us or prevent us from breaking a social or family rule.

"That's interesting. What else can I choose going forward."

Day 19

What family or social rules are you ready to break?

We maintain family rules because they keep us connected to our family. Are your family rules maintaining healthy connections?

We keep social rules because we don't want to feel silly or stupid. Have the difficulties in your life that caused you to create little boxes for important enough for you to resolve that you are willing to risk someone disapproving of you?

What is so important about your self-identity that you need everyone to approve of you? A great freedom you can give yourself is breaking free of the need for public approval. You can't please everyone.

Where are you holding yourself hostage to other people's standards? Do those people and their opinion really matter to you in the grand scheme of things? Would you be happier without those people in your life? Are you ready to reclaim your freedom?

I've talked to many married friends lately who said that if they were to get married all over again, they would do it completely differently. They sacrificed so much of what they wanted their wedding day to be like to accommodate other people.

If you have been sacrificing your life to accommodate other people, you can make the choice today to choose differently.

"That's interesting. What else, even greater is possible here? What other choices do I have? What would I decide to do if I didn't care what other people thought of me?"

Day 20

How much stuff did yesterday's questions bring up? I want you to know that it is a lie that you can't go against a family rule. That is a limitation that you and no one else is imposing on you. It's a lie that you can't choose something that other people might disapprove of.

You may have many things on your list right now that you might want to choose, but you tell yourself that you can't choose because of family rules or social norms.

At some point, you have to start being yourself otherwise you may end up looking silly anyway. At one of the restaurants I worked at, the owner was raised by a very conservative mother. When the daughter got her belly button pierced as a teenager, her mother prayed that it would get infected and have to be taken out. When the daughter (as a 35-year-old adult) decided she wanted to get botox in her lips, she explained their new size to her mom by saying that she had walked into a door.

I want to encourage you to quit judging your ideas. Quit judging yourself. You might look at your list of ideas and come up with a myriad of excuses why any one of them won't ever work. That won't get you anywhere. You've got to move through it and choose what is right for you.

Ask the question, acknowledge when you get ideas, write them down, and continue to ask the question again.

"If I didn't care what other people thought of me, what else would I choose?"

Day 21

Where have you been stifling yourself to keep fitting into this little box you created that you don't actually fit in? The more you stifle yourself in one area, the more it will bleed over into others.

Have you ever asked or thought, "Who am I being right now?" If you were actually being you, would you choose what you are choosing right now?

My husband and I don't argue a lot. Recently, we were arguing on a regular basis, once or twice a week, which is quite a bit more frequent than normal for us. I was very unhappy but didn't know what to do about it.

Finally, one evening, as we were heading down the argument road again, and I began expressing my frustration with it, Daniel said aloud, "This isn't us." By acknowledging that, the spell was broken.

We both regularly make the choice to listen to the other and are always finding ways to improve our relationship. We would never make the choice to tear it down.

Where have you made the choice to quit being yourself and began tearing things down that you would rather build up? What choice will you begin making instead?

Day 22

Do you even know what you want in your life? Have you defined it enough that you know what you don't want as well?

One of my favorite actresses played a role in the movie Runaway Bride. In the movie, she had no clue who she really was or what she liked down to even how she wanted her eggs cooked. When she got in a relationship, the way the man liked his eggs cooked become her favorite as well until they broke up and she got in a different relationship. Then her favorite eggs shifted to reflect the new relationship.

She couldn't commit to a relationship because she never honored herself or even knew what she wanted. Each relationship was just a new box to fit herself in.

When she finally began working towards her goals and dreams, she was able to have a healthy relationship.

Where have you hid what you actually would like from yourself in order to make others happy?

I encourage you to write down five things you desire your life to be, have, or feel like and five things you don't. You can't ever get what you desire if you haven't defined what that is.

Day 23

Imagine walking into a restaurant that has every kind of food imaginable available for order. You sit at a table and a server comes by to take your order. When asked what you want, you respond, "Food".

"What kind of food?" the server asks.

"I don't know. I'm starving. I'm very picky. I want some food."

This is another scenario for what we talked about yesterday. If we don't ever decide what we want, define it, and order it, we'll be disappointed with what we get.

The food server in this situation may bring you a basket of bread. How can they ever bring you what you truly desire unless you ask for it?

Think about the situation you are focusing these 30 days on. Write down five specifics that your optimal choice would be, do, have, feel like, or include. Then write down five specifics that your ideal choice would not include.

Day 24

"What is right about this situation that I'm not getting?"

Have you ever gotten ready for work and realized that the clothes you had planned to wear weren't clean? The next best option you can think of to wear needs ironed. You scramble to find something to wear and run out the door a minute late. On your way to work, you past the scene of an accident that happened a minute prior. You realize that if the first outfit had worked, you may be the one involved in the accident.

Too many times, we only look at what we think is going wrong in any given situation. Try asking, "What is going right here? What about this is actually working for me? I'd like more of that. What choice surrounding this would give me more of that?"

Day 25

Start noticing when you can't genuinely feel happy for the good things happening to others around you. This is often called jealousy. We see a co-worker get the raise we wanted and begin to wish them ill for it. Or a sibling gets a new truck while you still drive an unreliable junker. Sometimes we don't get what we want because we are unwilling to ask for it.

When I was about twelve, I borrowed my older brother's Bon Jovi cd's. A week after I returned them, my sister had them to keep. She had expressed her desire for them, and our brother had given them to her. I was jealous because I had discovered them first but had never told my brother how much I liked them.

I'm not implying that you should go around asking people for their possessions, but you should be asking yourself, "How can I get more of that in my life?" regarding things you would like.

Remember, your brain can go to work to help you figure things like this out while your body is resting.

Do you get enough rest in order to allow your brain to work for you?

Day 26

How many questions do you ask? We discover the world with questions. We learn about others by asking questions. As soon as children can talk, the questions pour out until someone makes them feel wrong for asking too many questions. You purchased this book because you were looking for a solution to your health problems. We can't find an answer to a problem until we ask a question.

Many professionals will tell you that there is no cure for autoimmune conditions; I'm telling you that the cure resides in you and your ability to support your body in every facet of health: physical, emotional, and social.

Ask yourself, "Do I believe that there is no cure for me and my health will continue to get worse OR do I believe that my body has the amazing gift of regeneration if I am willing to work with it?" Which questions gives you a feeling of lightness around it? The one that feels lighter is the truth for you.

Question everything, follow the truth, and keep asking, "What can be even better than that?"

Day 27

Do you find yourself sitting in and dealing with bad moods and negative emotions indefinitely? Have you ever asked if there is a different choice you can make?

It isn't wrong to feel negative emotions, but you don't have to sit with them forever. Feel them, acknowledge them, and then ask them to move on. Notice the word "motion" inside the word "emotion"? The origin of the word "emotion" dates back to 16th century France and means to "stir up" or "move out". Are you allowing the emotions you don't want to feel to "move out"?

The next time you experience a negative emotion, ask, "Do I really want to feel this way?" If the answer is "no", ask, "What could I choose to help this emotion move out?"

We always have another choice if we choose to ask for it.

Day 28

How many positive changes have you seen since you started this 30 day process? Once you open your ability to choose and change, your life can begin to contain more of what you want and less of what you don't.

Many people get stuck in frustration, fear, or guilt and never ask for anything better to happen.

With anything we are unhappy or dissatisfied with, we can ask, "What can I choose that would make this easier, better, happier, more satisfying, etc?" This can begin to loosen up situations that seem to be stuck.

We can ask the question when things are going well or great, too. Good things can always get better.

Day 29

What are you going to do about it? Anything worth having requires action to acquire. We can't say we want something different while remaining exactly as we are. Hopefully this 30 day exercise has begun to open up areas in your life that were stuck or trapped in a lie. Remember that lack of movement leads to stagnation and decay.

Negative emotions slow us down and lead to depression (stagnation) and inflammation (decay).

I hope you are ready to begin taking greater action towards what you desire more of in your life.

Day 30

In the early days of my husband's and my personal training careers, we had a client I'll call Emma who trained first with myself and then with my husband. Emma remarked to Daniel that everything he and I talked about doing together would actually happen and happen quickly.

I was the first of the two of us to get excited about becoming a personal trainer. Within one calendar year, we were both certified and owned a small fitness studio. At the fitness studio, we were unhappy that our business would stop making money completely if we needed a day off as we were the only two people working there. When we began asking how we could keep making money without physically needing to be present at the location, someone told us that the local 24-hour gym was available for sale. Because the members gained access to the gym via personal key cards, no one had to be physically present at the gym at all times.

By going after what we wanted, and then asking how it could be better than it was, we solved the problem of losing money if we took a vacation.

Years later, we problem solved how to allow people to purchase their membership online, further reducing the need to be physically present at the gym to increase our income.

All of these questions and ideas presented to you over the course of the last 30 days are tools that you can keep using to improve anything in your life. Just like an onion, the more you use them, the more layers you will discover that will keep opening up bigger and better opportunities for you in your life.

I hope that you will decide to continue with them and even repeat the process again and again.

We'd all love to hear how it has improved your life in the support group. (Find the link here: BookBonuses.NHWarriors.com)

13

Build: Providing the tools

Have you ever tried to make a cake and realized that you were missing some key ingredients?

Growing up, my older sister loved to make coffee cake on Sunday mornings. It was a decadent, sugary treat cause she tripled the part of the recipe for the crumb topping, which was essentially sugar, butter and cinnamon. Bits of it would carmelize in the oven. It was wonderful, and we often fought over the corner pieces.

Quite often, though, we would be missing an important ingredient that you can't make a cake without such as flour or eggs.

We lived outside city limits, and the closest grocery store was a fifteen-minute drive into the city. Fortunately, we had some amazing neighbors who lived just around the corner from us. Several times a year when we were out of something important for our coffee cake we would run over and ask to "borrow" a cup of flour or an egg or two.

Of course, we never really paid it back, and they didn't mind. One morning, when my sister and I knocked on their front door, the dad answered and immediately put his finger up to his mouth telling us to be quiet. He had just helped his wife deliver their sixth child at home. We had arrived minutes after the birth. In the gracious nature of that whole family, he still obliged us by getting the cake ingredient we were needing.

In the same way that we can't make a cake without all the important ingredients, your body can't make healthy cells unless it has all the ingredients of a healthy cell.

Do you know what is required for healthy bones?

The answer is not calcium. Can you make a strong building foundation out of just loose rocks and nothing else? That wouldn't be very stable.

Our bones are much more complicated than a building foundation. They are made up of protein and over 84 different minerals with new trace minerals being discovered all the time. We haven't even fully discovered every element that makes up our bones.

We need those minerals to be in an organic form, which means they are made up of living matter. Living matter in food (enzymes) is killed any time it is heated above 130 degrees Fahrenheit.

This means that all food that is pasteurized, cooked, or canned is now inorganic. It is much less beneficial to the body beyond satisfying calorie and macronutrient (fats, proteins, carbohydrates) needs. This is how we are overfed and undernourished in America. Our calories are devoid of the nutrients we need.

Just finishing up the strong bones conversation, pasteurized milk is not a source of organic calcium that our bodies can use. The structure of the calcium is changed during the pasteurization process to a form that acts as a toxin in our bodies that we can't process. Now, it has to be stored someplace in the body.

The most common kidney stones are made of calcium. Calcium contributes to cataracts and gallstones. It can accumulate in soft tissue areas and harden the arteries.

Many of my clients with plantar fasciitis respond well to a program designed to dissolve calcium deposits in the body that includes hydrangea and a good source of magnesium.

There are so many cases of bones fracturing that aren't caused by a lack of calcium but rather a deficiency of another needed nutrient. Healthy bones are 50% protein by volume. When we are protein deficient, there is nothing to bind the minerals together, so the bones begin to weaken.

Protein is a toxin when not digested correctly and can't be used for bone building. If you recall from the discussion on digestion, we need a highly acidic environment in the stomach in order for protein to be broken down into a usable form.

The vast majority of people have an under acidic stomach rather than too much acid, as we are commonly told. They take acid reducers which further perpetuate their poor digestion issues.

I start all my clients on a digestive enzyme supplement to take with every meal containing protein, whether that is animal or plant-based protein, that includes Betaine HCl, bile salt, papain, lipase, pepsin, and amylase to help them break down their foods and digest them.

Sonya's Story

When I first began working with Sonya, her face was literally ghost pale. I'm a very white person, and I joke that my skin is see-through. Sonya had me beat.

She was struggling with a winter cold and had a very difficult time concentrating as we talked. In fact, she attempted to write down every word I said as we went so that she could follow along and retain it. I hadn't ever seen someone in such a poor condition still carrying on with their life and multiple jobs.

We got interrupted halfway through our first meeting, and Sonya had to leave, but she had learned and retained enough information and began to apply it.

I was shocked about six months later when she came into the store and looked completely different. Her face had color; her eyes looked alive. She was retaining information. She scheduled an appointment with me and didn't even have to put it in her phone or write it down.

Sonya just recently celebrated the birth of her third grandbaby. With all the improvements in her health, she'll be able to thoroughly enjoy her grandbabies. Here's a bit more about her story and what had contributed to her pain issues.

Sonya's biological mother left her with an abusive stepdad when she was five. She struggled with feeling not good enough. Why else would her mom abandon her? She was in several less than ideal foster care situations after that. She never felt like anyone cared for her while she was growing up.

She ended up living on the streets sleeping on park benches. She was raped and became pregnant. She started her pregnancy at 98 pounds, and because of gestational diabetes and other unhealthy habits, she was close to 200 pounds when she had her baby.

A month and a half before her due date, she developed placenta previa and had to have an emergency cesarean.

Sonya wanted to be healthy for her daughter, but didn't know how. She started an unhealthy cycle of yo-yo dieting to try to get her weight under control. This continued through a second pregnancy.

After several abusive relationships, Sonya met an amazing man, and they were married in 1995. Being in a long-term, healthy relationship made Sonya even more desperate to regain control of her health and weight, but it was a losing battle.

One day, she drew a hard line in the sand for herself and her family. She had reached her heaviest weight ever at 298 pounds and was at her limit. She said if she reached 300 pounds, she didn't want to live anymore.

It wasn't just the weight that was making her life miserable. She had been off and on medications for diet and diabetes. She had a low thyroid diagnosis and was on medication for that. She was dealing with anemia, endometriosis, fibromyalgia, suspected rheumatoid arthritis.

Even on an extreme pain medication regimen, she would lay on the floor of her house bawling at times from the pain. One of her doctors even told her that all her problems would go away if she would just lose weight: fibromyalgia, diabetes, depression, etc.

Even at 298 pounds, Sonya wanted to be healthy and physically active. She became a Zumba Fitness Instructor while at her heaviest weight. In the room full of skinny fit girls, she got quite the looks, but she made it through a full day of strenuous training. She kept up with them all because she was determined and loved dancing. Deep down, she knew she was capable.

Even now, at every Zumba Fitness class that she teaches, she tells people,

"It doesn't matter to me how you move as long as you're having fun and you're out there moving, that's all that matters to me."

She was still concerned about her own ability to keep up with life. As a way to control her weight and help herself have a desire to live, she underwent gastric bypass surgery. She had already failed at so many other diets, including doctor assisted plans that included vitamin injections.

It took her five years of research and talking to people who had undergone gastric bypass surgery inorder to make the decision. This included people who had the surgery, lost a lot of weight, and gained it all back. Sonya was not going to let that be her story.

After the surgery, Sonya felt that there was a huge lack of viable nutritional information needed for her to take care of herself, recover, and lose weight. When she spoke with me, she realized that there wasn't an emphasis on taking care of our microbiomes. No one talked to her about gut health.

"Taking care of the gut. Wow, that's significant." That's what began Sonya's journey back to health. She realized that all the pain medication she was on wasn't fixing the problem. They weren't helping her heal; they were just covering up the problem. Even with all the pain medication she was taking, her pain level was still a seven or eight most of the time.

She says now that she didn't realize how much the medications were making her sicker. You can't realize that until you get away from it.

When I met Sonya, her pain was still so bad that she slept in a recliner and needed her husband's help to get up in the morning. He'd have to start her body moving and lift her out of the recliner.

She'll be the first to tell you it's a journey, and it takes a little experimenting in order to find out what will work best for you. She tried several different supplement combinations before finding what really would help her pain levels.

Here's some of the things she had to say when I interviewed her about her journey.

"But what's amazing about that is once you start this, you're going, 'oh wait', I can get up out of the chair and I haven't had any pain medicine. My husband hasn't had to lift me out of the chair. Or I've made it through teaching back to back Zumba Fitness classes five days a week.

"It's not that I immediately felt what those things (supplements) were doing, but I can immediately tell when I don't have those in my system now, which is a huge shift.

"It's kind of the difference between managing your quality of life and improving your quality of life.

"My plan is not to revert back to the old habits. My plan is to continuously challenge myself to regulate emotionally. Live in the now. Because this is a whole new beginning.

"And if you take every day as a brand new beginning and start from where you currently are, it makes a huge difference. If you constantly worry about the 'what if's', you can't continue to move forward. You can't enjoy the things you should be enjoying.

"My mom left me when I was five. But, I have an incredible husband of thirty years now and a new grandbaby.

"So my plan was and continues to be working with Tirzah and working within myself and challenging myself to help other people because this stuff has made an incredible life-changing difference for me.

"There are stumbling blocks. There are times when you're not going to make good decisions or you're in the midst of stuff and you might eat the wrong things and you might say the wrong things and you might look the wrong way for the occasion, but you know what? You just dust it off and you keep moving forward. That's it.

"This is coming from somebody who didn't want to live.

"It works and it makes a difference and it takes time. There's no magic cure and there's no quick fix. I didn't gain all that weight overnight. I didn't live the first 40 years of my life overnight.

"I'm pushing towards being the best version of myself that I can. And work with Tirzah, cause she's awesome.

Sonya just recently reached her two-year mark of being prescription free. (Dec 2019)

Key Learning

Your body and bones require over 84 different minerals.
Cooking food above 130 degrees Fahrenheit destroys all the enzymes in it.
Protein requires a highly acidic environment in order to be digested.
More people have too little stomach acid instead of too much.
Taking care of her gut helped Sonya with her diabetes depression, fibromyalgia, and pain issues.
It doesn't matter where you are starting from as long as you start.
Write down any other key points you would like to remember.

14

Cleanse: What does this mean?

A lot of people come into my retail store and ask me for a cleanse. Maybe they just got back from vacation or they want to lose weight or for some other reason. But they want to "do" a cleanse.

When I show them the box cleanses we carry, they ask what they can and can't eat with the cleanse. Do they need to start it on the weekend or will they be able to do the cleanse while working?

All these questions remind me of how much misinformation is out there concerning cleansing. Many people think cleansing means they are going to drink something nasty, fast for a day or two, and be stuck on the toilet for hours.

All of that is definitely not the correct way to cleanse.

I do promote the use of boxed herbal cleanses of ten to fifteen days at the beginning of each change of the seasons, but the need for cleansing goes deeper than that.

Let's talk a little about the boxed cleanses first. A cleanse of this sort needs to work with the body. Taking something that makes you feel ill is not working with your body. That is releasing toxins faster than they can be eliminated. This quite often happens when someone hasn't gone through the first two stages of activate and build before doing a cleanse.

When someone feels ill on a cleanse, I recommend slowing the cleanse and taking fewer toxin eliminating herbs. Your body can only process and release toxins at a certain rate. How quickly we can detox is determined by how many pathways in the body are open, how many nutrients are available for the detoxing processes, and the toxin load of the individual.

There is no need to be miserable by trying to detox faster than your body is able to. If you are already in a state of detoxing faster than your body can eliminate, doing a series of enemas can be helpful for flushing out some of the toxins that were stirred up and opening up an elimination channel.

A cleanse should not leave you glued to the toilet for any length of time. The point of a cleanse is to produce more bowel movements with a greater quantity to them. Most herbal cleanses contain some fiber that absorbs certain toxins and supplies bulk to the stool for cleaning the walls of the intestines.

If your stool is less than solid, you are flushing out water and electrolytes and not doing much to clean out toxins, which is the point of the cleanse. This is a sign that the cleanse is too harsh, or you are taking too much of it, or it doesn't contain enough fiber.

Cleansing is an Everyday Thing

Are you ever done brushing your teeth? At what point can you say, "That's it. That's the last time I have to brush my teeth. I've brushed them 10 times in my life. I think that's enough"?

Think about everything else in your life that you are never done taking care of: gardening, mowing the lawn, taking out the trash, washing dishes, taking showers. I'm sure there are many more you can think of.

We clean things that are much less important than our health on a daily basis. Why don't we practice the same care for our bodies? We only get one body. We can't go out and replace it the same way we can our car if it breaks down.

A garden requires weekly and seasonal maintenance. And during the summer it requires daily watering. Our body is a much more complicated living environment than a garden. Why do we neglect it so?

Just because our body has systems whose entire jobs are waste management and removal, why do we think they don't ever need care and upkeep? What is there in life that continues to improve without someone paying attention to it?

When we neglect our bodies, they will continue to deteriorate. If we don't clean our house frequently, it falls into a messy chaos.

We need to be focused on incorporating cleansing on a small scale into our daily habits and also targeted and seasonal deep cleansing the same way you would "spring clean" a house.

Do a google search for how many new chemicals are created each year and how many chemicals humans have created. It's really alarming when you research it because we don't know what kind of damage each one can do to our bodies.

Couple that with the fact that there are many natural invaders bombarding our immune system each day. Whatever the body can't process, it stores. Major known storage sites are fat deposits, bones, and the brain.

Many times, people yo-yo diet because they have too many toxins stored in their body fat. As they accumulate more toxins than their body can deal with, their body will create more storage space (fat) as a safe(er) place to put it than allowing it to circulate in the body.

When they lose their initial weight, the toxins are released, but the body still can't deal and process them. Also, most diet food does not support a healthy microbiome. The person has done nothing to change the actual health of their body, and the weight returns. The more unhealthy the diet food they ate, the more likely they are to put on more weight than they lost.

If we don't change the internal environment of the body and support it with a healthy lifestyle, then any diet is doomed from the beginning.

A lot of heavy metals are stored in the bones. Aluminum has an affinity for the brain where it contributes to Alzheimer's. For many reasons, heavy metals are not able to be removed by normal body waste disposal systems, and we are exposed to them on a very frequent basis.

Heavy metal toxicity is something that needs to be done slowly and over a great length of time.\

For more on heavy metal toxicity concerns see:
https://www.ncbi.nlm.nih.gov/pmc/articles/PMC4427717/

Key Learning

A "cleanse" should work with your body and not leave you miserable for a couple of days.

If we want to maintain the health of our body, we need to practice maintenance cleansing on a daily basis.

Many toxins are stored in our fat. We can't burn the fat without releasing the toxins.

Write down any other key points you wish to remember.

15

Cleanse: getting out the "bugs"

There are many pathogens and toxins that can contribute to our ailments. They weaken body systems allowing other infections to flourish. Some of these include viruses, bacteria, parasites, fungi, and heavy metals.

Viruses can contribute to chronic fatigue, chronic pain, vertigo, tinnitus, fibromyalgia, cystitis, Hep C, liver toxicity, lupus, Graves, Hashimoto's, nerve pain, muscle pain, joint pain, back pain, tingling or numbness in the hands and feet, migraines, dizziness, insomnia, night sweats, rheumatoid arthritis, menopausal symptoms, anxiety, heart palpitations, multiple sclerosis, adrenal fatigue, shingles, frozen shoulder, TMJ, and depression. This is not a complete list.

Bacteria can contribute to acne, chronic fatigue, diabetes, fibromyalgia, Hashimoto's, inflammatory bowel disease, irritable bowel syndrome, leaky gut, non-alcoholic fatty liver disease, obesity, abdominal pain or cramping, food intolerances, neuromuscular disorders, rosacea, and skin rashes. This is not a complete list.

Parasites can contribute to recurrent infections, unexplained constipation, diarrhea, gas, inflammatory bowel syndrome, difficulty sleeping, skin rashes, hives, rosacea, eczema, grinding of the teeth, painful muscles or joints, fatigue, depression, apathy, hunger after eating, iron-deficient anemia, anxiety, mood swings, Hashimoto's and Graves. This is not a complete list.

Fungal and yeast infections can contribute to chronic sinus issues, vaginal yeast infections, frequent colds and flu, earaches, swollen lymph nodes, fatigue, brain fog, leaky gut, athlete's foot, jock itch, food sensitivities, food allergies, nail fungus, sugar cravings, gas, bloating, indigestion, brain fog, and mental confusion. This is not a complete list.

Heavy metals can contribute to ADHD, autism, depression, rheumatoid arthritis, chronic fatigue, type I diabetes, fibromyalgia, lupus, Lou Gehrig's disease, myasthenia gravis, multiple sclerosis, cancer, heart disease, dementia, Alzheimer's, poor immune function, mental illness, and parasitic infections. This is not a complete list.

When I begin working with a client, I plan to address each of these over the course of the first year or two. I don't start with any lab test to confirm or deny any of these infections because many of them won't show up through many of the current testing methods. If someone has one or more of the possible symptoms of one of these infections, I'll start them on a protocol and notice if any of their symptoms go away.

The vast majority of people I've worked with have needed to address all five possible infections.

Vicki's Story

When Vicki first came to see me, she was dealing with memory issues, brain fog, nerve pain in her legs, muscle twitching, poor digestion, urinary tract issues, and just overall feeling drained. She wasn't even 30 years old and had two kids and a husband she wanted to be healthy for.

Her doctor wasn't offering many solutions. He was going to refer her to physical therapy and was considering MRI's to diagnose her with Multiple Sclerosis.

I recommended some supplements, including ones targeted at reducing a possible viral overload in her body, and encouraged her to stick with them for about nine months.

Now, Vicki has no more nerve pain and great improvements everywhere else. She has taken some of the knowledge she learned from working with me and applied it to help her kids be healthier, too.

Key Learning

Pathogens in the body can contribute to a wide variety of diseases and symptoms.
    We need to work on a continual basis to keep our pathogen load low.
    Write down any other key points you would like to remember.

16

Your Personal Consultation

The following is a list of questions that I use to go over with my one on one clients. Take the time to write down your answers in a journal and include the date. Then you will be able to go back in a month or two after following the suggestions in this book and answer them again to see improvements.

After each question, I will provide an explanation of the importance of the question as well as what a healthy answer should look like. As you continue to work on improving your health, you'll see your answers begin to look similar to those found here.

First, take a moment to write down your biggest health concerns and how long you have had them. These can be symptoms or diagnosis that are worrisome or troublesome to you. I ask my clients to prepare these in advance of meeting with them.

As you write them down, think back to when it started and write the circumstances surrounding that as well as how long you have had the concern for.

General Information

Don't forget to take the time to write your answers to the questions in a journal so that you can reflect back on that at a later date and note progress made.

How long have you been without great health?

The longer someone has been without great health, the longer it will take to regain it. However, I expect my clients to begin to notice improvements and a reduction in their number of health symptoms within a week or so of working with me. While it may be a journey to get rid of the issues you have had the longest, your health will begin to return as soon as you begin to pay attention to it. It can keep improving as long as you continue. There is no upper limit to how good you can feel except for those you create with your beliefs.

How long are you willing to commit to your health?

A good rule of thumb is to expect to dedicate one month for every year you have had a problem. If your thyroid has been struggling for two decades, then it will take approximately two years of eating correctly, supplementing what your body (whole body, not just the offender) needs, and lifestyle changes to get it back functioning as it should. For some people, it may take longer; for others, it may be shorter. It depends on how many roadblocks are in the way.

Ideally, you will never quit improving your health. At each stage in your journey be willing to ask, "How much better can this get?" and be ready for the answer to surprise you. Just like a property that you keep improving, your health can always keep improving if you keep paying attention to it. Whatever we tend to flourishes; whatever we neglect dies.

What is your current weight? Are you satisfied with it or looking to gain or lose weight?

No matter whether you are underweight or overweight, following the Natural Health Warriors program will help bring your body into balance. Many of the reasons for weight issues, whether over or under, are the same. I help my clients address all of these issues that may be connected to their weight.

What is your current blood pressure?

One of the most common causes of high blood pressure is a deficiency in magnesium. Taking additional magnesium to the point of bowel tolerance can help correct this. There are many other benefits to getting enough magnesium as well.

What is bowel tolerance? It means that you have comfortably loose stools. Too much magnesium acts as a laxative. Rather than taking one large dose of magnesium, I recommend breaking it down into two or three smaller doses for optimal absorption.

If stress is a contributor to your high blood pressure, I would recommend magnesium (the most common mineral deficiency) as well as taking a flower essence blend appropriate to your current personality needs and an adaptogenic herbal blend to help your body deal with stress in a healthy way. For a link to a quiz that can help you determine the flower essence blend most helpful for you, see the bonus book resources: BookBonuses.NHWarriors.com

What is your current cholesterol?

Cholesterol is highly debated between the Western medicine world and the natural health world. The brain needs cholesterol in order to function. Our body can't make estrogen, testosterone, and other essential hormones without it. Every cell in our body requires cholesterol as part of it's cell membrane, which controls what can go into and out of the cell.

While I won't argue that we need to keep bad cholesterol low, it is only harmful when it is oxidized. Cholesterol oxidizes at night; we can prevent this by taking a strong antioxidant formula before we go to sleep. Eating large amounts of organic fruits and vegetables can supply additional antioxidants.

Three-quarters of the cholesterol found in our blood was produced by our liver. This is why it is more important to address whole-body health for controlling cholesterol than by just looking at what we are eating. Foods only contribute one-quarter of blood cholesterol.

Cholesterol is needed to produce bile for the breakdown of fats in our diet. Eating lots of healthy fats as well as supplementing with flaxseed oil and omega-3 essential fatty acids can help to lower cholesterol as more bile will need to be produced to digest these foods thereby consuming excess cholesterol.

The body uses cholesterol to make vitamin D from sunshine. People with lower levels of cholesterol may find themselves lacking Vitamin D, even if they are out in the sun all the time.

In general though, for a healthy brain, healthy hormones, and healthy cells, we need healthy levels of cholesterol: 200-250mg/dL.

Resting pulse. Take your pulse after you have been sitting peacefully for about ten minutes.

When I was volunteering for a drug study a decade ago (before I was introduced to natural health), my pulse would be taken each week when I came in for monitoring. Several times they would remark at my fitness level or wonder if their equipment wasn't working properly because my pulse would often read as low as 52 beats per minute.

The current acceptable range for a healthy resting pulse is really too high in my opinion. You may hear that anything up to 80 beats per minute is acceptable. I prefer that my clients keep theirs much closer to 60 beats per minute if not below it.

My husband's grandma was in the hospital for bowel issues (I always say, "Constipation kills".), and the doctors were concerned about whether or not she was going to pull through during a dire time. They said it was all up to whether or not her heart was strong enough. My mom-in-law assured them that gma's heart was strong as she'd never had any issues with it. The doctor replied, "Does she get regular exercise that makes her heart work on a frequent basis? The heart is a muscle and needs to be worked."

If your pulse is too high, you may just need some exercise in your life. Are you keeping your heart strong and healthy by working it? Exercise helps the heart and body learn how to use oxygen more efficiently so that the heart doesn't have to beat as often.

Consider this: if your heart is beating 70 beats per minute when it could be beating 60 times a minute, that is 600 extra beats per hour and an extra 14,400 beats per day. What does that look like over a week? An extra 100,800 beats. How many extra a year is that? How many years have you been alive? You do the math on that one. Healthy hearts require exercise.

There is no excuse for not being able to exercise. When I owned a fitness studio with my husband and was leading dance fitness classes, I would go into retirement facilities and help the residents exercise while seated even if they were in a wheelchair.

Emotional issues and anxiety can contribute to a higher resting pulse than desired too. For these, I utilize adaptogenic herbs, flower essences, and emotional clearing.

Do a spit test. Three days in a row. Record the Results

Yes, this one often grosses people out. First thing in the morning, before you eat, drink or brush your teeth, spit into a clear glass container that has a few inches of water in it. The container needs to be clear so you can see what the spit does. Check it after about five minutes. Does it float? Sink? Get little jellyfish legs?

Healthy saliva sinks to the bottom of the glass. If it floats or has little tendrils coming down from it like a jellyfish, you may have an overabundance of candida in your body.

Candida is a nasty little fungus that can cause lots of problems in the body. Taking antibiotics won't affect it: they only attack bacteria. We can use natural antifungals to address candida. These are generally safe and help bring the body into balance.

Many women will get yeast infections following a round of prescription antibiotics. This is because yeast and bacteria are constantly fighting for space in the microbiome (gut). When we kill the bacteria (antibiotics kill the good with the bad), yeast and fungus can proliferate.

Candida can contribute to many symptoms and illnesses in the body including adrenal issues, allergies (food and environmental), asthma, athlete's foot, brain fog, chronic fatigue, cystitis, depression, earaches, fibromyalgia, frequent colds/flu, gas/bloating, irritable bowel, leaky gut, migraines, PMS, sinus issues, swollen lymph, vaginitis, yeast infections, weight gain, and so much more. I'm not sure the list ends.

Have you ever had so many symptoms and no one knows what is wrong with you or how to help you get better? Have you ever been told, "It's all in your head?" It's probably all in your gut. And quite frequently, addressing candida can help mystery symptoms disappear.

How does this all get out of balance? It's not just antibiotics, though they are usually one of the first offenders and frequently overused. Immune suppressing drugs shut down the immune system against these organisms. Being on birth control pills for longer than six months upsets the body's natural balance. (Who do you know who has been on birth control pills for LESS than six months?)

The Standard American Diet (SAD) makes another great contribution with all the refined sugar, refined flour, processed foods, and GMOs that we consume.

Stress and an emotional imbalance weakens the immune system. You'll find stress and emotions play a much larger role in our health than anyone ever told you before.

If you have candida, what can you do? Addressing yeast requires a five-fold approach.

Stop feeding it. What you quit feeding dies, right? We need to eat a low-glycemic diet for several months. You can find the first 30-day food list at the beginning of the chapter on the Natural Health Warriors program. I would recommend following it for at least three months if you suspect that you have candida.

Improve digestion and address possible leaky gut. Undigested foods rot and ferment in the body. What eats rotting and fermenting foods? Mold and fungus. I recommend that my clients take a food enzyme supplement with every meal. You can take a special protease formula between meals to help balance the microbiome. It will literally eat or digest unwanted things there. Candida and a leaky gut go hand in hand. Most people don't make progress if they aren't addressing both. I recommend taking l-glutamine and some strong natural anti-inflammatory supplements.

Kill the yeast. I've worked with many people who come to me after following an anti-candida diet for up to a year or more who still deal with yeast issues. Cutting off its food supply is only half the battle. You need to fire some rockets at it too. In the book resources, you can find some of the tools I utilize against candida.

Bring in good bacteria. Remember that bacteria and fungi compete for space. We need our microbiome to be about 80% good guys with only about 20% bad guys. We can keep the bad stuff at bay if we outnumber it four to one. The problem is that most people have the opposite ratio. We can repopulate with probiotics, but then we need to adopt eating habits that help good bacteria grow. Getting in plenty of fresh fruits and vegetables is really important here.

Elevate your emotions. I worked with a client who didn't begin to eliminate candida until we started doing some emotional work. Candida and parasites can't thrive if your emotions are too low. Those really low emotions are where the big C and death begin. The range above that is great for supporting candida and other bad bugs. We have to keep going up and get into better feeling emotions and then the body can naturally fight the candida.

As with every other symptom you may be dealing with, it's crucial to address the body as a whole and get all its parts working together again.

Basal Body Temp Test. Take three days in a row one week away from your cycle.

Directions: put a thermometer by your bedside. Before you get out of bed in the morning, record your temperature. Under your tongue is sufficient.

I consider this test a much more reliable gauge of how your thyroid is working than any blood test. Many people who receive normal reports on their blood tests will have an abnormally low basal temperature. This is an early warning sign of a struggling thyroid. Anything lower than 98 degrees Fahrenheit is too low.

Often, in addition to a low basal temperature, people will have many other symptoms that can be a sign of a poorly functioning thyroid. These may include sensitivity to cold or always having cold hands and feet, a swollen puffy face or eyes in the morning, excessive weight with an inability to lose weight, difficulty getting up in the morning and feeling tired when at rest, and excessive fatigue.

I recommend that anyone with a low body temperature begin taking herbs that feed the thyroid such as dulse, kelp, bladderwrack, and black walnut. These herbs are really good sources of organic iodine. I recommend herbs much more often than individual nutrients because each herb contains a wide spectrum of nutrients. Often, our body requires one nutrient in order to utilize the nutrient we are deficient in. These combinations are quite often found in nature.

The conversion of T4 to T3 takes place in the liver, another organ that needs iodine for proper function. If we have a thyroid problem, we usually have a liver problem as well. In general, I think of any organ or gland problem as a whole-body problem. It makes it easier to fix when we look at the whole body instead of just a small part. What good does it do to change a headlight if the car alternator is dead?

How much dental work have you had done? How many heavy metals are in your mouth?

Heavy metals can cause so much damage to our bodies. They are a major factor in autoimmune disorders such as rheumatoid arthritis, chronic fatigue, type I diabetes, fibromyalgia, lupus and other diseases such as heart disease, dementia and other mental illnesses. Candida and parasites flourish in the presence of heavy metals. You may not be able to get rid of one without getting rid of the other.

Did you ever wonder where the term "mad as a hatter" came from? Hatters, people who used to make hats, used mercury in some of their processes. This literally drove them insane. Yet, until quite recently, it was normal practice to store mercury in people's mouths. Open up yours and see if you have any silver fillings. Those contain mercury which releases anytime you chew your food.

Mercury isn't the only danger of traditional dentistry. Root canals, implants, crowns, bridges, braces all introduce heavy metals into the body. The wider the variety of these metals in a single mouth, the greater the damage they can cause.

We need to go to a biological dentist in order to have heavy metals safely removed from our mouth. There is a free packet about toxic dentistry and what questions to ask a dentist that you can send for. Find the link in the book resources: BookBonuses.NHWarriors.com

Just another word about heavy metals here: dentistry is not the only source of heavy metals in our bodies. Water is often contaminated. Food and supplements from certain countries often contain them. Cookware. Aluminum foil. Lead crystal. Even contact lens solution. The ink used for newspapers, books, and tattoos. Vaccines. Iodized salt and baking soda that doesn't say "aluminum-free" on the label. The antiperspirants found in deodorants.

In addition to getting toxic dentistry removed by a biological dentist, we should be taking herbs on a daily basis that are able to bind these metals and remove them from the body. A good heavy metal protocol will include specific herbs, antioxidants, binders, and essential fatty acids.

How many bowel movements a day? What is their consistency, color, odor, quantity or volume?

Constipation kills! I have a cousin who had to have part of her colon removed as a child and now uses a colostomy bag. My husband's grandmother almost died because of constipation. My own energy levels were sapped when I wasn't eliminating properly. This is a really serious wide-spread issue.

We should have a bowel movement for nearly every meal and snack we eat. Eating too often bogs down the intestinal tract. Limiting eating to a smaller window during the day can really help. Don't eat a large meal right before you go to bed. Get enough water. I think I covered most of this earlier in the book. Go back and reread that if needed until you understand the importance of having regular, productive bowel movements. So much ill health starts here.

Do you ever strain or feel like you wish you could go more after your bowel movements?

This is a sign of constipation to some degree and should be cause for a course correction.

How much water do you drink on a daily basis? What is the quality of that water?

Some people consume a lot of liquids while not consuming much water. When I was growing up, my dad rarely drank anything except for Pepsi and coffee. He ended up getting kidney stones.

My rule of thumb for my clients is an ounce for every two pounds of body weight per day up to about a 100 ounces a day.

The quality of your water matters. Some people who have a difficult time drinking water are responding to the toxins in the water. Your body knows if something is harmful for you. Invest in a quality filter and use glass drinking bottles.

How frequently do you urinate? Is there ever any pain or burning during urination?

If you just recently started drinking more water, I expect that you will be running to the restroom on a frequent basis. However, the more properly hydrated you are, the better your body will be able to use and store water.

Have you ever forgotten to water a potted plant until the soil had completely dried out? When you went to water it, the liquid ran off the top of the soil instead of being absorbed. The same thing happens when we allow our internal environment to dry out by not drinking enough water each day.

Personally, even if I get all my water in for the day, I still don't use the bathroom more than once every two hours or so.

How often do you get up at night to urinate?

Getting up once during the night is perfectly fine. Getting up more often than that is a reason to think about providing the adrenals some support. The adrenals are two little glands that sit on top of the kidneys. ("Ad" means above and "renal" means kidney.) They are responsible for turning the kidneys off at night. If this isn't happening, then I typically recommend something to support them. Adaptogenic herbs and B-vitamins feed the adrenals.

How many hours of sleep do you get a night and what is the quality of that sleep?

Sleep: so many people try to live without it. It doesn't take much sleep deprivation to start impairing your cognition and fine motor skills. If you think you are thriving on little sleep, you are just fooling yourself.

Sleep is not a luxury, it is a necessity. Difficulty sleeping is a sign that your body is struggling. Something isn't working right if you can't fall asleep and get six to nine hours of sleep a night. There are very few people who need less than eight hours of sleep at night.

Sleep is when your body does repair. It's when fat is metabolized. If you are trying to lose weight and not giving your body time to sleep, it can't get rid of the fat. It does that while you sleep.

Do you ever notice how your phone or your computer runs slow when it needs to be restarted? Your brain needs a nightly reset. This is when your body does its house-keeping. The brain is cleaned out while you sleep. Don't neglect your sleep while expecting your body to get better.

Do you have difficulty falling asleep or do you have trouble staying asleep?

One of the first thing I recommend for sleeping difficulties is magnesium. After that, I may suggest an herbal formula containing passionflower, valerian, and hops. This blend is great for anyone who's brain won't shut off at night, too.

Your sleep hygiene also needs examined. Are you drinking coffee after lunch? Are your adrenals stressed to the point where they don't know how to turn off to allow you to sleep? Disturbed dreams are another sign the adrenals need support.

If you commonly wake up between 1am-3am, that is a sign your liver may need additional support.

Do you go to bed at the same time each night? Do you get up with the sun and get enough daylight each day? We need sunlight in order for the body to know when to wake up and when to go to sleep.

Trying to go to sleep after doing something stimulating can be detrimental. Looking at a screen that puts off a blue light like the television or your phone before bed can delay melatonin production.

I don't often recommend melatonin to my clients. I would rather work with them and their body to find out why it isn't producing it's own.

An unhealthy microbiome can lead to sleeping difficulties. Melatonin is made from the neurotransmitter serotonin, which is mostly produced by a healthy gut. When the gut isn't healthy, not enough serotonin is produced, leading to a lack of melatonin.

How often do you feel rested in the morning?

Some people sleep but don't feel rested when they wake up. Typically, I will recommend thyroid and/or adrenal support for these instances.

I never used to be a morning person. Even after ten hours of sleep, I'd have to drag myself out of bed in the morning. This still happens from time to time when I'm not taking as good care of myself as I should. But in general, I can tolerate an early morning alarm much easier now. I don't prefer mornings, but they are definitely easier the healthier you are.

How often do you experience low energy?

Low energy from time to time should be expected. We can't just go and go without taking a rest. Low energy on a daily basis is definitely a sign that the body is missing something it needs or is overburdened with toxins.

In this case, I start by looking at what the person is eating. Are they taking digestive enzymes with their meals to be sure they are getting the nutrition from it?

Next, I look at how much water they are drinking. The body runs off of an electrical current that needs water in order to conduct that electricity. Our body is mostly water, or at least should be.

Not exercising will cause someone to frequently have low energy as well.

Exercise also improves circulation, and good circulation is necessary to distribute oxygen throughout the body.

After I've looked at all that, I will then look to see what needs there are for supplements to supply nutrients or help the body clean itself out.

Does your energy level drop in the afternoon?

There are three things that come to my mind first when I hear a "yes" response to this question.

Digestion is difficult work. Your body is reserving energy to digest your lunch. Eat a lighter lunch and take enzymes with it.

Sugar or caffeine crash. If you ate something earlier that spiked your blood sugar levels, they may be dropping now. Depending on the state of your digestive system, liver, and pancreas, even whole carbohydrates and protein can cause this spike. Also, if you use caffeine to get you going in the morning, then I would expect a crash from that. We want to support natural, all-day energy instead of consuming one stimulant after another.

Your adrenals may be exhausted. No matter the cause, the body is tired. We just need to find out what is missing in order to have even energy all day long.

How is your memory?

We all have days where we forget things, and stress just exacerbates that sometimes. Memory is something we can practice. It doesn't help if we tell ourself that we have a poor memory. The mind takes that as a sort of order, and will follow our expectations. Start telling yourself that you have an amazing memory; you remember more important things each day, and that your brain is improving in health. Then consider these needs of the brain.

The brain needs oxygen. I have a favorite drink mix I take that helps dilate the blood vessels in the body, including those that supply oxygen to the brain. It definitely is a favorite of mine for waking up in the morning, helping me workout, and improving blood flow at any time of the day. It helps increase nitric oxide in the body like nothing else out there. Of course, you can learn more about it in the book resources.

B-vitamins are essential for brain health. I found enough information on how important B-vitamins are for brain health, mental health, and memory that I was able to write a fifty-page dissertation about it.

Alzheimer's is being called type three diabetes or diabetes of the brain. Too much sugar and refined carbohydrates in the diet negatively affects the brain. Blood sugar spikes are the equivalent to eating too much sugar. Even if you aren't diabetic, you can still monitor your blood sugar levels to see how different foods affect you.

Don't forget that the brain also needs sleep as discussed before.

How hydrated are you? The brain is 70% water. Being one or two percent dehydrated will be enough to start negatively affecting brain function.

Good fats. Don't think of all fats as a four-letter word. There are some that are essential to our health. That's why omega-3 is called an essential fatty acid (EFA). The brain needs healthy fats for proper function. I recommend several (at least 3) tablespoons of healthy fats a day. Refined fish oil, olive oil, coconut oil, olives, avocados, etc.

Clean out the toxins. Heavy metals accumulate in the brain. We need to slowly and safely help the body eliminate them.

Do you have difficulty gaining or losing weight?

Yes, I have met people who want to gain weight. They often end up feeling as self-conscious about their lack of weight as people who have too much do. Often, these people can eat as much as they can force down and not gain an ounce.

I always go back to digestion and the gut in these cases. Even if you have low levels of thyroid hormones, the thyroid issue started someplace too. Usually the gut. Our weight is a whole body issue. We need to address it as such.

How much exercise do you get? How many days a week? Hours a week? At what exertion level?

When I ask this question, the most common answer is "not enough". Exercise is one of the best, free things we can do to boost our health, yet so many people are averse to it. We tell ourselves we don't have time, or it hurts too much, or it's too difficult. Everyone can exercise. Even if it is from a chair.

You can find exercise videos on YouTube for any fitness level.

List your allergies. Include food, environmental, and anything else.

There are three reasons why we get allergies. Personally, I believe that no one should be allergic to anything that is natural. We should not be allergic to dogs and cats, grass and trees, and organically grown foods.

It was bad information from the beginning. When I was growing up, my mother had a lot of chemical sensitivities. The pastor's wife at the church we went to was such a hugger, but she wore perfume that made my mom's head and body hurt for about 24 hours after exposure. Eventually, my mom just quit going to church because the perfume and detergents that people used and came to church smelling of were too much for her. If she went to church at all, she would often spend the rest of the day at home in bed.

People who are allergic to food may often be allergic to the chemicals in that food. A friend of mine can't eat blueberries. They make her break out in a rash. However, she started using a meal replacement shake from the supplement company I use with all my clients that contained a little blueberry powder in it. She was unaware of this for months and was able to use the supplement without issue.

The same thing happened to a colleague's wife. She was deathly allergic to watermelon; it would cause anaphylactic shock. But because the supplement company we use with our clients does such a thorough job of testing their ingredients for pesticides and other toxins, and will reject materials if they don't meet the rigorous testing requirements, she was able to consume a supplement containing watermelon without issue.

Food and everything else coming into contact with the body through our five senses is information for the body. If you are bringing in faulty information, such as chemicals, pesticides, and toxins, then the body will react to it with an error message. Sometimes we are reacting to the chemicals in the food instead of the food itself.

We need to evaluate the information coming in any time we are getting an error message from our body. In this case, an allergic reaction could be one of many different error messages.

Our digestive, intestinal, and hepatic system are bogged down. I'm sure this was another contributing factor to my mother's strong response to chemical perfumes. With her diet and lifestyle, none of those key systems could be working correctly.

One of the biggest differences between people who have strong reactions to chemicals such as perfumes and those that don't is the health of their liver. A healthy liver will be able to cope with exposure to some chemicals though we should take care not to overtax it.

Food can quickly become an allergen if it is not digested properly. Strawberry ice cream contributes to strawberry allergies in children because of this. Fruit does not digest properly when it is eaten with fats and proteins. These partially undigested or even fermented fruit components are then absorbed into the body and the blood stream. The body recognizes them as a harmful invader and launches an attack.

Taking a complete food enzyme supplement with meals can ensure proper digestion of foods to eliminate the possibilities of this happening.

When we support our digestion, clear out a clogged intestinal system, and address the liver, we can eliminate allergens to healthy food.

Our emotions created an allergic response to something we perceived was a danger. Jane could trace her dog allergies to starting right after she had a traumatizing experience with a dog. Her body took the information about a dog that it received from all her senses and noticed the panic hormones her body was producing. Therefore, her body perceived canines as physical threats. Whenever she was around something that carried dog information her body would attack the information as a dangerous invader. We would call it an allergic response.

When she began to utilize different emotional healing techniques, and neutralized that trauma she was carrying around, she was suddenly no longer allergic to dogs. This same process can happen with environmental allergies and foods.

A note about celiacs disease. I have heard of people with celiacs reversing their allergic response to gluten enough that they can eat organic ancient grains such as spelt. I'm not sure that someone with celiacs would ever get to the point that they can eat conventional wheat and similar products because the gluten in those foods is a toxin to the body. It's not something natural that the body was made to process. Today's hybridized wheat has thousands of times more gluten in it than ancient grains because it makes it fluffier and helps it last longer on the shelf.

Occupation and Recreation

List all the jobs you can remember.

I ask clients this so we can evaluate if and how their work history might contribute to toxicity in their body. There are many jobs that someone may have where they are breathing in fumes or particles. It's quite common in people who develop asthma or lung problems.

After you list all the jobs you have held, evaluate whether or not they may have been a source of toxins in the form of chemicals, viruses, bacteria, parasites, emotions, people, etc. Those all leave an impact on the body that needs cleared.

List your current occupation and how many hours a week you work.

Are you working too much?

How do you feel about your current job?

Is your current occupation a source of joy in your life? Does it contribute to the life you want to have? Do you feel good when you go to work? If you work with people, do you feel a sense of gratitude that they are in your life? Do you feel that they are grateful for you?

If your current occupation or lack of current occupation is not contributing to your ideal life, I would encourage you to use the 30 Day Process included in this book that helps you change things in your life that don't contribute or bring joy to you.

Travel history. Where in the world have you been?

Similar to your job history, your travel history provides some insights into whether or not you may have traveled to some place where you could have picked up an exotic bug or parasite. Whenever I travel, I always supplement with black walnut as it is a wonderful anti-parasitic herb. Just remember, you don't have to have traveled out of the country in order to pick up a parasite. We are exposed to them everyday. I recommend seasonal parasite cleanses as a maintenance program.

List your favorite hobbies, activities that bring you joy and how often you engage in them in the average week.

You are the one who gets to decide how much time you spend doing things you love. Do you make room for joy on a weekly basis? A daily basis?

Always remember that you have to put on your oxygen mask first before you can help others. If you are not joyful then you are not able to contribute joy to others' lives. What emotions are you contributing to others'? The emotions you live in are part of your contribution to those around you. Are you teaching your children, friends, neighbors, how to take care of themselves by the example you set?

You deserve time to do things that bring you joy. If that brings up blocks for you, you may want to journal and apply the 30 day challenge to this area of your life.

How many close relationships do you have? Who are they?

I define "close" as anyone you can truly be yourself around and be accepted.

We all need relationships that allow us to be our true selves. We can't hide ourselves from everyone. That just brings in more unhappiness. The lack of someone who accepts us as we are and everything we are can be a contributing factor to depression. Begin to cultivate relationships in which you are accepted for who and what you are.

For some people, just having one or two close relationships is enough. Others need more. Make time for these people by not giving as much time to people and activities that bring you down. You have the power to make this choice everyday. Don't give away your power. Don't give away your choices.

How often are you with the people you are close to? Is this enough time for you and your mental health?

We need to be around people we can be ourselves with on a regular basis. Some people need this every day; some only need it once or twice a week. Evaluate how happy and fulfilled you are with the amount of time that you spend with people who you are close with. Is it enough? What can you choose if it is not?

The 30 Day Challenge may be helpful here. We get locked into thinking that we only have one or two choices in any given situation. This is because your conscious mind is only presented with your most common choices by your subconscious mind. Keep a list of things you want to use the 30 Day challenge to change and go through it as often as necessary. Remember that you have a whole group of people cheering you on when you participate in the challenge in our online group. Find the link in the book resources: BookBonuses.NHWarriors.com

Mental Health

Are you able to turn off your mind?

A lot of people have minds that run away from them. They can't turn them off or shut them up. One question you could ask when your mind is going on and on would be, "Is this mine?" We pick up other people's thoughts from the emotions they give off. You may find that this helps quiet the voices to ask the question. Another great question would be, "Is this contributing to me?"

An easy way to know if the thoughts you are thinking aren't yours is if they talk to you using the word "you". "What are 'you' doing?" "Why did 'you' do that?" If we are truly talking to ourselves, we would ask "What am 'I' doing?" "Why did 'I' do that?"

Many times the accusing voices in our heads are things we heard from our parents, peers, co-workers, etc. We don't need to hear them over and over again. Just acknowledging that the thought isn't yours is enough to help silence it.

If it is your mind going on and on and it would be helpful to slow it down especially so you can relax and sleep, I would recommend using a blend of herbs containing GABA, l-theanine, and/or passionflower. These can all contribute to calming overactive brain chatter.

GABA is a calming neurotransmitter that the body can naturally produce. Most neurotransmitters are produced in the gut. Any time the brain has a deficiency in an important neurotransmitter, we need to address and balance our microbiome. Following the protocols presented here will help with that.

List your traumatic experiences.

You get to decide if an experience was traumatic for you or not. If it had a lasting negative impact on you, your body, or your psyche, I would consider that traumatic.

When I was five years old, I was in charge of feeding our bunnies. The bunny food was kept in our pump house, which was a dark and scary place for me. One day, when I was getting the bunny food, a spider fell on my head. I screamed and shook it off; but for decades, my heart would race whenever I had to go into a similar space as our pump house. This wouldn't have been traumatic for everyone, but it was for me.

Be sure to list physical traumas as well such as car accidents, surgeries. Include emotional traumas such as abuse or the loss of a loved one or thing. Anything that you can think back on that upsets you and you feel a negative physical response such as increased heart rate or sweaty palms about was probably a trauma.

All traumas are a stress on the body and weaken our immune system. Some people find that their health began to deteriorate after being in an accident. For others, it was being in an abusive relationship. You need to list all your traumas and go through the process of releasing the emotions surrounding them. Just because you went through something horrible doesn't mean that you should carry around the horror of it in your body. You'll know that you have healed the emotions around a trauma when you can look back on it without any negative physical or emotional reactions.

For some people, removing the emotions from a trauma will relieve the physical pain or ailment in the part of the body that is carrying that trauma.

We can pick up traumas from an early age, even from when we were in the womb. We can inherit them from our parents and grandparents. If we were unwanted as a growing being, that can be a trauma we carry with us that leads us to believe that no one wants us. This is a lie that we can let go of if we choose. Are you ready to release your traumas? You have the choice.

For those who are working with releasing traumas of an emotional or physical nature, I highly recommend taking a flower essence blend that helps people dealing with distress. Be sure to utilize it regularly, meaning every day, for at least three months.

Flower essences help to break up emotional patterns in our body. The longer you have had the trauma and the more intense it is in your body, the longer I would recommend staying on the distress blend. It is also helpful for children who suffer from night terrors.

How often do you live in sadness, anger, anxiety, and/or overwhelm?

We need to evaluate what emotions we are living in. The longer we spend in the lower emotions, the easier it is for us to stay there. These emotions become habitual, and we can become addicted to the way they make us feel.

This doesn't mean that we shouldn't experience them. We just need to limit how long we allow them and set an intention to feel more love, joy, and peace in our lives. Being happy is a choice we can make and a good habit to cultivate.

Imagine your teenager sneaking into their bedroom two hours after curfew. When you confront them, they say, "I was just with my friend" or "I forgot the time". What is your response? Usually to get angry. Why? Because you know they are lying. One of the biggest sources of anger in our lives is when we are faced with a lie.

Think about that the next time you are angry. It's okay to be angry. For a short period of time. Acknowledge the anger; let it pass; then ask, "What is the lie here?" Ask that when you get angry and you will start to get answers. And they may surprise you.

Also, anger issues can point to toxicity in the liver. Using something that can help the liver balance is really helpful to the point of finding a completely new calmer person underneath all the anger. I utilize liver formulas for anger issues; adrenal formulas for overwhelm and burnout, and mood formulas for sadness. These are all in addition to balancing the microbiome.

I once heard "When we are depressed, we are living in the past. When we are anxious, we are living in the future. When we are happy and content, we are living in the present." Based off of that, where are you living and where would you like to live?

How high is your stress level? How well do you feel you handle stress?

Many people live with high levels of stress and cope with it very well. They don't mind having multiple balls in the air; they juggle them with ease and still live happy fulfilling lives. It's when we don't handle stress in a healthy way that there is an issue.

We can't avoid stress, but we can equip our body with nutrients to help us handle it in a healthier way. For this purpose, I would use a targeted flower essence blend based on the person's specific circumstances, adding magnesium to bowel tolerance, and providing support for the adrenals. Adaptogenic blends are great for this.

Are you able to relax? How often do you relax?

I once heard the idea that Sabbath observance was a rule instituted for man's benefit. We all need time off. Our body has limitations and requires rest. Many workaholics are unable to even take a few hours off. Work on incorporating something relaxing into your weekly, then daily life. This can be as simple as sitting in silence and relaxing for ten minutes a day.

How is your libido?

All of our bodies were made to produce sex hormones. Except in the case of trauma and abuse, we should all have a healthy sex drive. An inbalance in our sex hormones can lead to a lack of a libido. While there are herbs that can help balance our sex hormones, I find that correcting our hormones through our diet and lifestyle is a deeper, longer lasting solution than just taking a male or female blend of herbs. I teach my clients how to use diet variation with intermittent fasting to optimize their hormones.

Do you struggle with infertility?

It requires a healthy body to make a healthy baby. Many people who struggle with infertility are so out of balance that their body knows it isn't wise to get pregnant. The best time to plan for a healthy baby is a year or two before you plan to get pregnant. The same goes for men and women. I would encourage anyone struggling with infertility to take some time to follow emotional and nutritional protocols similar to the ones in this book for at least a year.

The more toxins and deficiencies your body has, and the longer you were on hormone altering chemicals such as birth control, the longer it will take to bring your body back to healthy enough to carry a child.

By taking the time to strengthen your body and give it what it needs, the healthier your children can be. A baby growing in the womb picks up about 10 percent of it's mom's heavy metal load.

Were you delivered vaginally?

A baby's first inoculation is the one it gets from passing through a birth canal full of good bacteria. If the mother is deficient in good bacteria, then the baby's immune system is weakened from the beginning.

How much unprotected sun do you get?

So many of us slather our bodies with chemicals and then go out and let the sun bake them into our skin. When you put things on your skin, part of it gets absorbed. A good rule of thumb for skin care is if it isn't safe to eat, don't put it on your skin.

Vitamin D is the most common vitamin deficiency in North America. We are taught to fear the sun. I encourage you to do some research regarding chemical sunscreens and skin cancer as well as the link between low sun exposure and higher cancer rates in general.

We need the sun! Every spring, as soon as it is sixty degrees outside, I am out on my deck soaking up as much sun as I can. Where I live in Oregon right now, I can be out there for hours in March and not get burnt. Then, as the summer rolls in, I never need sunscreen to prevent burns because I built up my sun exposure. During the winter months, I become a real pale white, but not nearly as pale as I used to before I started getting as much sun during the summer as I could without getting burnt. Now, I make it a habit to utilize a tanning bed with at least 75% uvb bulbs each week when I am unable to spend enough time outside.

If I do get burnt, I take care of it that day. Utilizing an enzyme spray, high-quality lavender and peppermint essential oils, and natural skin care lotions, all except for the worst burns will become a tan overnight and never peel.

The best form of vitamin D is the stuff we get from the sun. It is not nearly as beneficial for us as taking a supplement. If you live above the 45 parallel of the earth though, the sun is never potent enough for us to get enough vitamin D. Vitamin D is fat soluble and can be stored for year round needs if you get enough of it.

Remember that you need cholesterol in order to synthesize vitamin D from the sun. We need to get over the idea that cholesterol is a bad word.

Now, because I live so far from really, truly hot sun during the summer, when my husband and I travel to the Carribean area on vacation, I'm going to take a natural sunscreen with me as there is no other way for me to enjoy my time on the beach and not get burnt. Natural sunscreens also contain antioxidants that help undo the damage. I keep my enzyme spray and essential oils on hand for any accidental burns that happen.

What compulsive behaviors do you experience? Include work, sex, rage, hand washing, phobias, relationships, addictions, thoughts and anyth ng similar.

Keep a list of all your compulsions now because you might be surprised when they start disappearing.

Growing up, I had a really strong fear of spiders. I remember being about twelve years old, standing in the auditorium at church, when my little brother ran up to me with a spider in his hand to scare me. I screamed, which made all the adults nearby think someone was being murdered.

This fear stayed strong and extreme until just a few years ago. I realized that when my adrenals are healthy and I'm dealing with stress in a healthy way that I don't have as strong of a reaction. It's a reminder to me, when I have an extreme reaction to a spider or a loud noise even, that my adrenals need some extra nutrients.

Not everything on this list can be attributed to stressed adrenals. Some of it may be associated with neurotoxins, deficiencies, trapped emotions, and more. The point is to keep track of what you are experiencing now and to what degree so you can see progress when you check back in on these questions in the future.

Diet

How many servings of raw fruits and vegetables do you eat per day?

I'm finding that more and more often, people are having a difficult time digesting raw fruits and vegetables. When they eat these, they often experience painful gas and bloating.

Enzymes are required for us to break down the foods we eat. Raw fruits and vegetables contain the enzymes in them needed for us to break them down. The enzymes in raw fruits and vegetables are the reason they rot and get mushy. They are being digested. Eventually they turn back into soil matter.

Think about a processed food that you can leave out on a shelf for months at a time that never spoils. This food is lacking enzymes. Enzymes are the keys to life. Any food lacking enzymes is essentially dead.

It's not so much the digestion that happens in the stomach with raw fruits and vegetables that leads to the painful gas and bloating after eating them. It's more common that we don't have the probiotics, good bacteria, in our gut to finish breaking them down. Also, we may have too much bacteria in our small intestine, where it doesn't belong, that leads to the discomfort.

Raw fruits and vegetables are good sources of fiber which is food for our good bacteria. If we have too much bacteria in the small intestine, and we eat fiber rich foods, it feeds that bacteria and allows it to further grow out of control. Also, we may be lacking the specific probiotics needed to break down certain plant parts altogether.

In these situations, I utilize a three-part approach:

Take steps to reduce the amount of bacteria in the small intestine. One of my favorite supplements for this is berberine. Berberine is a bitter alkaloid found in plants such as goldenseal, Indian barberry, and Oregon grape. It has very potent, natural antibacterial properties.

One of the biggest benefits to taking an herb with antibacterial properties is that it will only go after the bad bacteria in our body and leave the good bacteria alive and well.

Take a food enzyme blend that incorporates cellulase. This is an enzyme that helps to break down plant cellulose.

Slowly incorporate good probiotics. This may need to be done a month or two after including berberine in your supplement regimen if there is too much bad bacteria in the small intestine.

How many cooked fruits and vegetables do you eat in a day?

How much fruits and vegetables is enough? Raw fruits and vegetables are best because of the nutrients and enzymes lost during cooking, but cooked fruits and vegetables are still valuable.

I recommend about six servings of vegetables consumed daily. This can be a mix of cooked and uncooked. A serving is half a cup of finely chopped or packed vegetables such as diced onions, mushrooms, tomatoes, etc. or a full cup of loosely packed or whole vegetables such as broccoli florets or cucumber slices.

If someone is dealing with too much yeast or bad bacteria, then I will initially eliminate fruits from their diet while we work on correcting their body's balance of these harmful overgrowths. The sugar in fruits can impede their progress.

The easiest fruits for those recovering from yeast or bad bacteria overgrowths to begin incorporating back in are berries and apples. After most poor digestion issues are eliminated, I recommend two servings of fruit per day.

How many leafy greens do you consume in a day?

Leafy greens are some of our best sources of organic calcium and magnesium. I recommend five to six ounces daily.

How many raw nuts and seeds daily?

Raw nuts and seeds are wonderful sources of healthy fats. When we roast them, however, we change the molecular structure of the fats making them not so healthy.

Nuts and seeds can be difficult for people to digest, though. Some, like almonds, should be soaked before consuming. Seeds can be sprouted to make them easier to digest.

Please note that peanuts are not nuts; they are legumes and often carry mold. I suggest eliminating peanuts from the diet for the most part, especially if someone is dealing with a bacteria or yeast overgrowth.

How many grains do you eat daily?

A lot more people are aware of the benefits of eating gluten free than are aware of the benefits of eating grain free. Grains fall into the macronutrient category of carbohydrates. By definition, a carbohydrate is anything that breaks down into sugar in the body.

Sugar is one of the biggest sources of inflammation in the body. Even though complex grains break down slower than refined grains, the result is still sugar. This includes but is not limited to rice, wheat, and non-gluten grains.

I recommend excluding these until inflammation in the body is under control. After that, I recommend eating grains on a limited and rotating basis.

How much fish and seafood do you eat a week?

Fish and seafood are great sources of iodine and essential fatty acids in our diet. Iodine is an essential mineral for our thyroid and liver. Essential fatty acids like omega-3 needs to be consumed in our diet or supplemented.

I would suggest one to three grams of ultra-purified omega-3 supplements for someone who consumes fatty fish several times a week. For those who don't consume fish at all, I would suggest three to nine grams a day as well as a kelp or black walnut supplement.

How much dairy do you consume on a daily basis?

Contrary to popular opinion, pasteurized milk is not a source of organic calcium. Thinking that we can use calcium from pasteurized milk is like thinking we can suck on a rock and get usable calcium.

Our perfect source of organic calcium is leafy greens. Plants are made to absorb minerals from the rocks and soil and hold it in a form we can use.

Also, dairy contain lactose, a form of sugar. You can recognize sugars in foods as they usually end in -ose, such as glucose, sucrose, lactose, galactose, and fructose.

Because sugar causes inflammation in the body, I seek to eliminate as much sugar as possible from the diet. Therefore, I recommend reducing dairy consumption to a minimum.

Some of the best dairy-based foods are no-sugar added yogurts and kefir as long as they contain active live cultures.

As a rule of thumb, I recommend no more than six ounces of dairy-based foods or one ounce of cheese a day.

For anyone experiencing any of the warning signs for autoimmune, I recommend eliminating dairy completely for at least one to three months while working on repairing their microbiome.

How many meals/snacks a day do you eat?

Digestion is one of the most-energy consuming process the body does. This is why we often feel sluggish, lethargic, and sleepy after eating, especially if it was a big meal.

Most of us ask our body to maintain a steady state of digesting food all day long. I used to be a big promoter of snacking all day long as a way to maintain a high metabolic rate. Now I teach my clients a better way of eating utilizing intermittent fasting and diet variation.

However, for the first six months of my Natural Health Warriors protocol, I start my clients with three meals and two snacks a day. So many people are insulin resistant. We need to teach the body how to stabilize blood sugar levels or else they will feel miserable when they first try intermittent fasting.

When do you eat breakfast?

By definition, breakfast is the first meal you eat in a day. It has nothing to do with the time of day you eat it. In the first six months of the NHWarriors protocol, I suggest that a breakfast containing about 30 grams of protein be eaten within 30 minutes of waking up.

Many people who are used to eating sugar-filled breakfasts or skipping it altogether notice an increase in energy and brain function when they adopt this habit.

How often do you eat out?

There is very little nutrition found in the majority of food prepared for us at restaurants and fast food joints. When we want a healthy meal when eating out, we can choose two from the following components: low sugar, low fat, or flavor.

Processed and restaurant foods use a lot of fat or sugar for flavor. If you eliminate one of those, you often have to increase the other. Plus, the fat used in restaurant and fast food preparation is usually cheap and unhealthy.

The easiest way for me to avoid grabbing convenience food is to prepare a week's worth of food on the weekend. When my food is mostly prepared and easy to eat, I am less likely to eat something I'll regret.

My advice for eating out is to avoid cheap unhealthy food during the week and save your eating out dollars for a really nice meal that you and your body will thoroughly enjoy.

Do you ever get light headed between meals?

The most common reason for this is blood sugar fluctuations. When our body isn't working correctly, even protein-rich foods can spike blood sugar levels.

A spike in blood sugar is commonly followed by a crash. Eating low glycemic meals rich in healthy fats while working on diet and lifestyle changes to balance insulin responses are what I recommend to solve the issue on a long-term basis.

How often do you feel gas or bloating between meals?

This is often a sign that the digestive system needs some assistance. I suggest incorporating food enzymes with meals while working to strengthen your microbiome for proper food digestion.

How often do you experience heartburn or acid reflux?

Except for in the smallest percentage of cases, this signals a deficiency in stomach acid. The vast majority of people, contrary to popular belief, have too little stomach acid, not too much.

Drinking raw, fresh celery juice first thing in the morning can help to provide the organic sodium needed to make stomach acid. I also suggest adding a complete food enzyme supplement containing betaine HCl with every meal to help insure proper food digestion.

How often do you use antacids?

When we use an antacid, we are perpetuating our low stomach acid problem. It is better to use food enzymes and betaine HCl to bring up stomach acid to the levels it needs to be at for proper food digestion.

Recently, a correlation between antacid use and dementia and nerve damage is being studied.

Antacids work against natural body processes. I would rather work with the body for proper digestion.

If you have undergone a stomach acid test and are one of the few people who have high levels of stomach acid, I would recommend supplementing with fennel when you eat.

What foods disagree with you?

As you embark on your health journey, I expect this list to decrease. It is my opinion that we should not be allergic nor have an issue eating healthy, organic foods.

Have there been any recent changes in your appetite?

Have there been any recent changes in your thirst?

Many people mistake thirst for hunger. Older individuals tend to drink less water and are prone to dehydration.

If you have had a sudden increase in thirst, this may be a sign of blood sugar levels that are too high.

How much caffeine do you consume? Include coffee, tea, soda, and energy drinks.

Sustained, high levels of caffeine intake are very taxing to the adrenals. When this happens, even a cup of coffee can spike blood sugar levels.

I typically suggest a 30-day break from caffeine at the beginning of following the NHWarriors protocol. This includes black tea and colas. The purpose of this is to give the adrenals a break from constant stimulation while we are providing nutrients to help them rebuild.

Many people think that just because they are "used to" their multiple cups of coffee during the day that it doesn't affect their sleep. When the adrenals become burnt out, though, one of the first things to suffer is their sleep.

Do you depend on caffeine to keep you going?

This is another sign that your body and adrenals are overstressed and need a break. We can't maintain high levels of productivity without proper rest, down time, and nutritional support.

How much alcohol do you drink?

High alcohol use is considered more than one drink a day on average for women and more than two drinks a day for men.

Personally, I consider sugar just as toxic as alcohol. Too much sugar affects the liver just as much as alcohol does.

Do you use tobacco?

Smoking depletes the body of vitamin c which is needed in the body as an antioxidant and for the utilization of collagen.

Also, nicotine blocks the receptor sites of niacin, also known as vitamin b3.

Different Diet Types

Vegetarian/Vegan

I really don't recommend vegetarian and especially don't recommend vegan diets. I find that my clients who have adhered to these diets for a substantial length of time often are deficient in bone mass.

Protein is required for strong bones. Without it, the minerals have nothing to sit on. It is often difficult to get enough complete protein in a vegan or vegetarian diet.

The protein alternative for someone eating vegan/vegetarian is grains and legumes, both of which are carbohydrates. Remember that carbohydrates turn to sugar in the body, and sugar causes inflammation. Most of our health issues start because of inflammation in the body. Think of inflammation as a smoldering fire in the body.

I recommend that grains and legumes are removed from the diet for the first 30 days of the NHWarriors protocol and then eaten only sparingly afterwards. It would be very difficult if not impossible for a vegan or vegetarian to then get the protein needed for their body to repair.

Diabetic

The sole purpose of this way of eating is to help you live with a disease. My goal is that you work with your body and provides what it needs for it to heal itself.

AIP

I have had clients come to me after a couple of years of following the AIP (AutoImmune Protocol) diet. They are frustrated because this plan doesn't allow for you to add back in foods that aren't on the plan.

Excluding gluten, my goal is for my clients to be able to eat any food in moderation. There are some people, especially those who have dealt with a leaky gut, who may never be able to eat traditional gluten-containing foods again without doing a high degree of damage to their gut lining.

The biggest fault I find with the AIP is that diet alone is often not enough to correct the extreme health issues caused by today's poor food supply; busy, stressful lifestyles; and rampant health issues. We need to be taking quality, targeted supplements that help our body repair.

High Protein

High protein diets can lead to over acidity and place a strain on our kidneys.

For the first six months of the NHWarriors Protocol, I recommend getting in about 100 grams of protein a day. This is normally done by having 30 grams with each meal and about 5 grams with snacks. This typically results in an increase in bone mass, especially when the protein is digested properly with the use of enzymes and vitamin c is added to the supplement regimen.

Most of the protein used by the body is made by the body. Therefore, if we support normal body function, we don't need to consume additional protein.

Low Fat

Low fat diets contribute to poor heart health and inflammation in the body. We need to be consuming lots of healthy fats every day.

I promote staying away from toxic and rancid fats found on most grocery store shelves and opting for organic, cold-pressed oils such as olive, avocado, and coconut. We also need to consume more omega-3 EFAs than omega-6 in our diet. Omega-3s are commonly called marine omegas as they are often sourced from fish and seafood. Omega-6s are usually plant based.

Low Carb

Low carbohydrate equates to low sugar in my mind. When people come to me for advice about too much yeast or cancer concerns, I typically tell them to cut out all sugars including carbohydrates as carbohydrates turn to sugar in the body. This includes rice, flours, oats, grains (including gluten-free grains), and starchy vegetables such as white potatoes and corn.

The carbohydrates that you can eat with abandon are limited to non-starchy vegetables. I recommend eliminating the rest until most health issues are resolved and then limiting carbohydrates on an on-going basis.

Low Sodium

The sodium found in most processed foods is a toxin to your body, especially the irradiated 'iodized salt'. Natural salts, such as a real sea salt and himalayan pink salt, are full of minerals good for the body and are a better choice for cooking and eating.

The body needs sodium however, especially the stomach which utilizes organic sodium to make hydrochloric acid. Raw, fresh, organic celery juice first thing in the morning is an excellent source of needed sodium. Other rich sources are leafy green vegetables.

Gluten-free

The biggest issue with gluten is that our food supply is being composed of hybrid wheat that contains much more gluten than ever before.

Gluten is a protein, and proteins are some of the most difficult foods for us to digest because of the decreasing ability of people to make enough hydrochloric acid. Proteins are broken down in the stomach in a highly acidic condition. If we are deficient in stomach acid and can't create an acidic enough environment, proteins are not digested properly.

Undigested proteins are a big source of toxins, allergens and inflammation.

Most people who have had a history of leaky gut will need to avoid gluten for the most part because it is a big source of inflammation.

However, I have heard of instances where even people with celiac have been able to repair their gut lining enough to tolerate ancient strains of wheat that contain much less gluten than standard commercial wheat.

Medical History and Conditions

List any medications you are currently taking.

Make a list of the current medications you are taking and how long you have been on them. It is my goal for as many of my clients who want it to be able to discontinue the use of all their chemical medications.

The goal of chemicals is to stop a normal function in the body. I prefer to help my clients work with their body to restore health naturally. The end result of health is a cessation of symptoms.

However, please do not discontinue any of your prescriptions without working with your doctor.

There was a lady I was working with, I'll call her Trish, who decided on her own that she wanted to stop all her prescriptions. We had just started working together. Because she went through several chemical withdrawals at once, she was miserable for months. This was not an ideal, nor necessary, scenario. Some prescriptions have severe side effects when quit cold turkey.

Always work with your doctor concerning your prescriptions. As a drugless practitioner, I do not consult with people about their prescriptions, nor give any advice or make any recommendations concerning them.

What medications have you been on in the past?

It is helpful to make a list of past medications and the length of time you were on them for. This gives you an idea of some of the chemical burden your body is operating under or chemical damage that needs to be repaired.

A history of frequent antibiotic use can give insight into how damaged the microbiome of a person is. The longer someone was on birth control pills, the longer it will take for hormones to be able to balance naturally.

List your current medical conditions.

List the current medical conditions you are dealing with and how long you have been dealing with them. Remember that a good rule of thumb for health recovery from a condition is approximately one month per year that you have experienced the issue. The less dedicated you are to following all recommendations, the longer it can take for these to resolve.

List Past Medical Conditions, Illnesses, and Surgeries

It is helpful to know what diseases and surgeries someone has experienced in their past. For instance, someone who has had a hysterectomy will need to do additional work supporting their adrenals in order for hormones to balance naturally.

Someone who has had their gallbladder removed, will have a more difficult time digesting fats and should supplement with additional lipase when they eat fatty foods.

Someone who has had their tonsils removed will need to do additional work supporting their immune system.

If someone has had mononucleosis, they may need to do additional work clearing viruses from their body.

Those are just a handful of things that past medical history can alert us to.

How often do you have headaches or migraines?

Most commonly, I suggest magnesium to bowel tolerance, as well as maintaining hydration levels as a good place to start for stopping frequent headaches.

Headaches associated with a woman's monthly cycle are usually stopped through balancing hormones and supporting the liver.

In general, most headache sufferers see a drastic decrease in the number of headaches they experience when they follow the NHWarriors protocol.

What is your monthly cycle like?

A natural cycle is about 28-30 days long and often corresponds to cycles of the moon. Cycles should never be ultra heavy. Also, I do not recommend skipping your period for any reason. It is a normal body process and should be worked with, not against.

Do you experience any PMS or menopause symptoms? Describe them.

Neither a woman's monthly cycle nor her time in menopause should cause more than a little discomfort. If it does, I recommend addressing stress, liver toxicity, and trapped emotions.

When I first learned about trapped emotions from the book The Emotion Code, I went through the process of clearing them from my body. I had already been working on my health naturally for about ten years at this point. I had been able to reduce my PMS symptoms through herbs and lifestyle changes, but I still had a day or two of breast tenderness, bloating, and abdominal cramping.

Once I finished the process of clearing my trapped emotions, my PMS symptoms abruptly discontinued. One month they were there; the next they were gone. I have no physical or emotional issues leading up to my monthly cycle now.

Prior to that, I used to have a day or two with extremely heavy bleeding to the point that I almost always bleed through whatever feminine products I tried overnight. Now, I have about twelve hours of heavier blood flow than the rest of the days, but it is considerable less than ever. And the days I bleed have reduced from seven to five. I would expect similar results for clients who address the cause of their hormonal imbalances.

I would recommend the same work for someone suffering from menopausal symptoms such as hot flashes and mood swings. Of course, all these approaches will work better if someone utilizes them before beginning menopause.

Do you ever get restless legs? Describe frequency and severity.

Before I started correcting my health, I used to get restless legs that were so painful. When I would try to go to sleep, I would roll onto my stomach and bang my legs against the bed as hard as I could.

Restless legs can be attributed to a lack or imbalance of electrolytes, poor circulation, or inflammation. Potassium, magnesium, and homeopathic remedies are helpful to ease the symptoms while you work on addressing the root cause.

Do you ever get cold hands and feet, especially when others are a comfortable temperature? Describe.

Cold extremities, especially when others around you are comfortable, can be a sign of poor circulation or a struggling thyroid.

How often do you experience muscle cramps?

Muscle cramp causes are similar to the causes of restless legs.

Do you experience any muscle pain, abdominal pain, back pain, joint pain, arthritis, or gout symptoms. Describe.

When someone experiences pain, doctors often diagnose them with a name ending in "-itis" such as arthritis, tendonitis, myelitis, etc. "Itis" means inflammation. The beginning of the word describes where the inflammation is located.

Taking large quantities of natural anti-inflammatories such as curcumin and omega-3 can help lessen the pain while someone works on reducing the cause of the inflammation in their body.

Like restless legs and muscle cramps, muscle pain may be attributed to a lack of electrolytes or not enough water.

Abdominal pain may have to do with a hiatal hernia, an inflamed ileocecal valve, too much bacteria in the small intestine, poor digestion, parasites, or a yeast overgrowth among other things.

Some muscle and joint pain can be attributed to a sedentary lifestyle and resulting poor circulation. The body needs to move. Consider the quality of water that is found in a stagnant pond where the water doesn't move and mosquitos and algae breed and flourish to that found in a crystal clear rushing river. Movement doesn't allow for parasites to breed and grow.

Gout is just a form of arthritis.

Do you experience any acne, rosacea, eczema, psoriasis, fungal skin infections, or other skin issues. Describe.

A lot of these just speak to the health of our liver and microbiome. Any external skin issue mirrors a similar internal issue.

What supplements do you currently take?

How many of these are from a big box store or a warehouse store? Collect these and put them in the trash. Many of these big brand supplements are more harmful than helpful. Some of them can't be broken down by the body and can accumulate in dangerous ways. You can find information about the supplements I personally use and recommend to my clients in the bonus area: BookBonuses.NHWarriors.com

 I am way more picky about the supplements that I take than even the personal and home care products I use. Brand matters. And I do believe with supplements, that you get what you pay for.

 Margret came into my retail store asking what I suggested for her digestive issues. She listed off the symptoms she was dealing with. When she was done, I walked over and grabbed my favorite brand of food enzymes and said, "This is what you need."

 Margret told me that she had already gone to another health store, and they had suggested digestive enzymes as well. She had paid $20 for a 90-ct bottle, and they weren't doing anything for her.

 I had heard of the brand she had bought before and was familiar with it. The previous owner of my retail store used to carry it, and I quit carrying some of the random, low-quality brands when I purchased the store.

 I asked Margaret to give my brand a try. It was comparable at $28 for a 120 count and had a one hundred percent money back guaranteed by the company. She could finish the bottle, and if she still didn't think it helped her, I could refund her 100%

 Margret purchased my recommendation and went home. She came back within days telling me what a night and day difference she felt between the brands. Whereas the cheaper brand did nothing for her that she could tell, what I had suggested had relieved her symptoms 100%. That is the difference value provides.

Personal and Home Care Products

What brand of deodorant do you use?

I recommend using a natural deodorant. If fragrance is wanted, choose one scented with essential oils.

Be sure not to use one containing an antiperspirant. Our armpits are a major dumping site for lymph. My mentor (who has been a natural health practitioner for 30 years) has noticed lumps situated between the armpit and breast are able to be dissolved and broken up just by discontinuing an antiperspirant. Many antiperspirants also contain aluminum, a dangerous heavy metal linked to Alzheimer's disease. I believe there is a link between using an antiperspirant and a rise in cases of breast cancer even in men.

What brand of body wash do you use?

Remember that what you put on your skin can be absorbed into your skin, your body's largest organ. We can reduce our toxic load by not using products on our body that contain chemicals. Skin care products should be safe enough to eat, though I doubt they'll taste good enough to eat.

There are some wonderful body washes out there containing magnesium. These are delightful to also use as a bubble bath. Some people have difficulty absorbing magnesium taken internally. When we use a body wash containing magnesium, some of the magnesium is absorbed through our skin.

Helpful ingredients to avoid include parabens (endocrine disruptors), phthalates (endocrine disruptors and cause liver and kidney damage), polyethylene glycol (carcinogen), sodium lauryl sulfate (aka SLS, skin irritant), and triclosan (linked to cancer and is also an endocrine disruptor).

What brand of shampoo and conditioner do you use?

If you want to check the toxicity level of any personal care item, you can search the EWG (Environmental Working Group EWG.org) database at SkinDeep.org. They provide toxicity ratings of personal care items and ingredients.

Some brands of shampoos contain gluten. This can cause issues for those with gluten sensitivities.

SLS (sodium lauryl sulfate) is often added to shampoos and body washes because it helps the product suds up. Many natural soaps don't have a big sudsing action to them. There are many studies on PubMed pointing to this product causing toxicity issues. I recommend avoiding it.

What brands of laundry products do you use?

Many laundry products are full of harmful chemicals and fragrances. These chemicals can be absorbed into our skin while we wear our clothes. The synthetic fragrances are not good for our lungs. There are some natural laundry products out there that work just as well and are scented with essential oils.

What brand of toothpaste do you use?

If you do not already use a natural toothpaste, check the box and see if there is a warning about swallowing too much of it. Why are we putting something in our mouth, where it will get absorbed directly into our bloodstream, if it's not edible?

Other stipulations I have for my toothpaste include being fluoride-free, sls-free, gluten-free, and paraben-free.

Did you know that fluoride is a neurotoxin? Yet many people still use a fluoride toothpaste, go to their dentist for fluoride treatments, and drink water containing fluoride. Fluoride is not good for the brain, especially for children's brain development. It may contribute to autoimmune conditions and negatively affect the thyroid and our bones.

Opt for a natural toothpaste containing essential oils such as tea tree and neem. I have had several customers at my retail store who saw an improvement in their teeth and gum health when they switched.

What perfumes and air fresheners do you use?

I grouped these two together because they are both made up of toxic fragrances. The best perfumes and air fresheners to use are ones made up of high quality essential oils.

List your face and skin items and brands.

Again, I don't put things on my skin that aren't clean enough to eat. Start evaluating everything you buy that touches your skin. It all adds up. Just like a single straw isn't responsible for breaking the camel's back, just one thing that you use or do isn't making the difference between health and disease for you. Little things add up.

I imagine if you are reading this far in the book that, like me, you don't want to be a workhorse in life carrying a huge toxic burden that weighs you down. This doesn't have to be done all at once. Just switch what you use from chemical to natural as you run out of personal and home care items.

Gradually it will begin to make a huge difference. You'll also notice how using a chemical really makes you feel and how your body was compensating because of it.

What brands of cleaning supplies do you use?

Isn't one of the first things people do as their child learns to crawl and walk is lock up their cleaning supplies? Why? Because they are so toxic they can kill someone. Every time you use those products you ingest them through your skin and breathe the fumes into your lungs.

If I asked you to carry a one pound rock around with you, that probably wouldn't be much of a big deal. Imagine that everything chemical in your house that you use is a one pound rock that you carry. This is the unseen burden you are placing on your body that contributes in small ways to the breakdown of your health.

Count the cleaners in your bathroom, the chemical products in your bathroom cabinet and your laundry room. How many little one pound rocks do you have adding up to a big burden on your health?

Now add a rock for each junk food item in your fridge and cupboards. Add a rock for every day you don't exercise or drink enough water or eat out. How big is your pile of rocks?

The cleaner I use for almost everything in my house except my toilet is made by the same company that produces the supplements I use. I mix an ounce of concentrate with about 32 ounces of water and fill hand pumps in my bathroom and kitchen and a general cleaning spray bottle. The general cleaner spray is used on every surface in the house that calls for a cleaner: counters, stove, sinks, floors, bathtub, etc.

It lasts forever, and it's safe. I can use it as a body wash and pour it into my bath water if desired, which actually is beneficial as well. A colleague of mine took a bath with a few ounces of the cleaner when she was experiencing a fever and felt that it helped her recover faster. It's already scented with essential oils that leave everything smelling fresh.

One day an elderly man called the company and asked if the concentrate cleaner was supposed to produce so many bubbles. Customer support was confused because a natural product like this cleaner doesn't actually produce a lot of bubbles when you use it. He said it was creating a lot of bubbles - out his butt!

He didn't realize that it wasn't a supplement and was drinking the concentrated cleaner. No one was worried though. It's not really toxic.

Now, I'm not saying to go drink it, but you probably don't have to call poison control if your child gets into it. Come to think of it, there isn't really anything in my house that I would be concerned about someone ingesting. Talk about peace of mind if you have kids around.

Do you have any new paint, carpets, bedding, mattresses, electronics, etc?

This is a good question to ask if you are suddenly feeling worse and don't know what to attribute it to. New products that contain synthetics and plastics go through a period of time of off-gassing when they are new.

One of the best ways to expedite this process is to place them out in the sun until the smell is burned out. Of course, it isn't possible to do this with new paint or wall to wall carpets. If you need to apply paint, try to do it during the summer when you can keep the room aired out and choose a paint with low or zero VOCs: volatile organic compounds.

Do you have houseplants?

There are quite a few houseplants known for removing all sorts of crazy chemicals from the air. Spider plants are one of my favorites and really easy to keep alive. They have been studied by NASA for their ability to clean the air.

A quick google search will provide you with about ten different house plants to choose from for improving the air in your home. I have them in several different rooms in my house.

Resources

You can find a list of suggested personal care products and a place to purchase them from in the member areas: BookBonuses.NHWarriors.com

Summary

That is the full consultation I used to go over with my clients on their very first visit. I understand that it can be very overwhelming, but there is a lot that needs to be covered in order to find where to start first.

I realized after going through it with people for over five years that I was suggesting the same protocol over and over again and making the same recommendations.

I hope you take the time to go over it and write out your responses to it again three months from beginning to follow the NHWarriors protocol. Look at it again at six months and again at one year. I have not had one client who stuck with the protocol for ever a couple of months who didn't experience drastic changes in their health.

The good news is that results can start quickly. Especially when you focus on digestion and the microbiome. Those are the hub of the body. If the hub isn't working correctly, then the rest of the body begins to have issues.

17

A 30 Day Food List

The full Natural Health Warriors protocol is based on a one-year cycle. The first three months are devoted to activating the body and opening up it's pathways. The second three months are focused on rebuilding the body and eliminating nutrient deficiencies. The third and fourth three months are about learning intermittent fasting, how to incorporate keto on an occasional basis, diet variation, and cleansing as a life-long process.

You can find a printable food list and sample supplement protocol in the complementary member's area for this book: BookBonuses.NHWarriors.com

Food list

Before I show you the food list for the first 30 days, I want to talk about the mindset you need to have around it. Many people will look at this list as restrictive. They'll examine the list and wonder or complain about their favorite foods that aren't listed.

A better attitude to have is looking at this list as a stepping stone to freedom. The goal is for my clients to become healthy enough that they can consume any food they want in moderation or on an occasional basis. Of course, there will be a small percentage of people that respond poorly to conventional gluten products no matter how infrequently they have them. It all depends on the strength of the constitution of your intestinal system.

The purpose of restricting the foods that someone eats initially is to eliminate common allergens and inflammation causing foods. If a body is constantly in a stressed state from fighting allergens or inflammation, it can't allocate energy for health and repair.

Once the 30-day period is over, clients in my NHWarriors program are given an expanded food list and taught how to reintroduce foods one at a time based upon a heart rate allergy test they can do at home.

Proteins

Water-packed canned fish
  Wild-caught fresh fish: cod, halibut, herring, Pacific salmon, pollack, sardines, sole, trout
  Wild game: bison, buffalo, elk, ostrich, venison
  Try to buy organic, grass-fed, pasture-raised versions of the following:
  Beef
  Lamb
  Pork
  Poultry: chicken, Cornish hens, duck, quail, turkey

Vegetables

Organic is preferred. If unable to purchase organic for all, then check the latest dirty dozen list and buy organic versions of the foods listed there.
  Artichokes
  Asparagus
  Bamboo Shoots
  Beets
  Bok choy
  Broccoli
  Broccolini
  Brussels sprouts

Cabbage
Carrots
Cauliflower
Celery
Chives
Cucumbers
Fennel
Garlic
Green beans
Jicama
Kale
Leafy greens (all)
Leeks
Lettuce
Mushrooms
Okra
Olives (canned in water)
Onions
Parsnips
Radishes
Scallions
Sea veggies (seaweed, kelp)
Shallots
Spinach
Squash (acorn, butternut, spaghetti, yellow)
Sweet Potatoes
Turnips
Zucchini

Fruits

Organic is preferred. If unable to purchase organic for all, then check out the latest dirty dozen list and buy organic versions of the foods listed there.

Apples
Applesauce (unsweetened)
Apricots
Avocados
Bananas
Berries: Blackberries, Blueberries, Strawberries, Raspberries
Cherries
Coconut
Cranberries
Figs
Grapefruit
Grapes
Kiwis
Kumquats
Lemons
Limes
Mangos
Melons
Nectarines
Oranges
Peaches
Pears
Pineapple
Plums
Tangerines

Healthy Fats

Avocado
   Avocado Oil
   Coconut Oil
   Grapeseed Oil
   Olive Oil
   Safflower Oil

Seasonings

Apple cider vinegar
   Basil
   Bay leaf
   Black pepper
   Cacao (100%)
   Cardamom
   Carob
   Cilantro
   Cinnamon
   Clove
   Coconut Aminos
   Coconut Vinegar
   Cumin
   Dandelion
   Dill
   Fennel Seed
   Garlic
   Ginger
   Lavender
   Mustard
   Nutmeg
   Oregano

Parsley
Rosemary
Sea salt
Tarragon
Thyme
Turmeric

Beverages

Water (preferably filtered)
    Herbal teas (unlimited)
    Green tea (if needed, in moderation)
    Fruit and vegetable juices (homemade, in moderation)
    I strongly recommend adhering to this list for a 30 day period at a minimum.

18

Thank You

Thank you for purchasing this book and taking the time to read it.

This book is really just the tip of the iceberg when it comes to repairing your health, but it is important for you to know and understand before moving forward.

This book is but the second one in the Natural Health Warriors Series. As I release each book, I'll also release a companion workbook to help you through the process. Please don't think of this book as ever finished. I plan on making many revisions and updated editions as necessary. You can help me in this process. Send me an email with your suggestions and any questions this book inspired: Tirzah.NHWarriors@gmail.com

If you found this book valuable, I would greatly appreciate if you would leave a review of it on your favorite ebook site or any other site that you purchased it from. This is one of the best ways for you to let others know of the value it provided you.

A positive review is the best compliment you can give an author, and I promise to read them all.

Please recommend this book to anyone you know that it may help. Let's spread health through the world, one person at a time.

I wish you much health and many blessings.

Look for the next installment of the NHWarriors Series to be released soon.

-Tirzah Hawkins

Also by Tirzah Hawkins BCHHP

I am on a mission to teach everyone who wants to learn how to become a Natural Health Warrior. Join the NHWarrior movement and look for future books in the series to be published soon (Spring 2020).

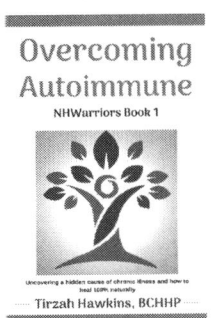

Coming Soon: Overcoming Autoimmune Book 1
Uncovering a hidden cause of chronic illness and how to heal 100% naturally.

Coming Soon: Natural Health Warriors Devotions
Have you ever wondered what truths about health and well-being the Bible holds?

Volume 1 contains 90 days of exploring the scriptures in short 5 minute devotions.

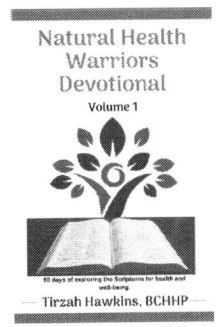

Made in the USA
Middletown, DE
14 February 2020